STUDENT NURSE, "60s STYLE"

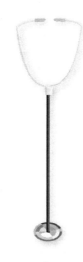

B. Park-Dixon

authorHOUSE®

AuthorHouse™ UK Ltd.
500 Avebury Boulevard
Central Milton Keynes, MK9 2BE
www.authorhouse.co.uk
Phone: 08001974150

First published by AuthorHouse 4/21/2009

ISBN: 978-1-4389-4758-7 (sc)

*Printed in the United States of America
Bloomington, Indiana*

This book is printed on acid-free paper.

All the stories in this book are based on true facts. The names of all characters have been changed, with the exception of Beryl and Ray.

CHAPTER ONE
1966

"Come on, B., open it up,"

said my impatient husband as I stared down at the envelope, wondering what the contents would be. I looked across at my baby sleeping peacefully in his cot, and then at the anxious face of my husband, who had sat across the table from me every night for the last few months firing questions at me, determined that I should pass my finals. My mind wandered back over the last six years to the end of my final year in school. It was quite sad, really; I actually liked school. I don't want to leave school. I knew what was expected of me, I knew the routines, and I guess I was in my comfort zone. There were just seven of us who had stayed on at school to sit for O'level. It was quite unusual to have a fifth form in a secondary school – usually it was only grammar school pupils who sat for O'level, but we were considered a bright class who would be able to work without supervision for some of the time.

Alfred Barrow was set right in the middle of town. When it was first built, it was the higher grade

1

school. By the time I went there, it was a secondary modern. It was divided in two halves; boys and girls were totally separated, and their paths never crossed. As our headmistress, Miss Black used to say, boys were just a distraction we could well do without. Miss Black would almost fly into morning assembly with her gown billowing out behind her and a mortarboard perched on her head. I'm almost sure she flew into school each morning, parked her broomstick on the roof, and slid down the chimney. She was always ready to preach fire and brimstone if she had spotted a girl looking into the boys' playground. Woes betide anyone who was seen actually talking to a boy. I think you were supposed to turn into a pillar of salt or something.

Being in a fifth form meant we were given lots of responsibilities. I was a prefect, the form chairman, and vice captain of my house. (I'm not too sure of that last title. I mean, the innuendoes are obvious, being the captain of vice, but I learnt to live with it.) The point is, I had loads of responsibilities. Although, naughty girl that I was, I actually broke a rule once. When the fashion was to wear little cat bells tied on the ends of the cords that ran around the bottom of your anorak (yes, anoraks were considered the height of fashion, and even more so with the little bells tied to the cords), Miss Black instantly banned them. She banned anything that was remotely fashionable. The bells were frivolous, but I left mine on. If I saw her coming, I would hold the tiny bells in my hands and pull the cords into my pockets so she couldn't hear them.

Anyway, it seems now was the time to move on, it was the end of my school years and the big, wide world beckoned. I was never one to shy away from a challenge.

It was with the utmost confidence that I went for an interview with a man from the Ministry of Labour, Youth Employment Office. This was a person who came to school just for the day in order to sort out what we would do for the rest of our lives. I went along to the library for my interview, and without hesitation, pushed open the door and strode in. I sat down opposite an overweight bald man who looked like his tie was about to choke him.

"Have you thought about what you would like to do?" he asked without looking up.

"Yes", I replied without hesitation.

"Well, what is it?" he asked as he looked over the brim of his glasses. I couldn't help but notice a slight irritation in his voice; it was nearing the end of the day.

"I want to work with animals".

"With animals?" He sounded almost incredulous.

"Doing what, exactly?"

"Well, I thought something like a veterinary nurse".

"A veterinary nurse", he repeated like a parrot.

He paused for a moment and then said,

"I'll tell you what. How about if I arrange for an interview at the hospital for a cadet nurse?"

As an educated female, it was presumed that I would either work in an office or as a nurse – girly things.

"But I really like animals", I said

"Try being a cadet nurse first, and if you don"t like it, you can always change later", he said soothingly.

I think he had had enough for the day and just wanted to get home. I became mesmerised by the way the light reflected off his bald head. I should have put my point more forcefully, but instead, I went into a daydream, hypnotised by the patterns the lights were making as he moved his head from side to side, muttering,

"Work with animals indeed".

And that was it. That's how I got into nursing. A couple of weeks later, I had gone along with my letter of introduction for an interview with the matron at the North Lonsdale Hospital. There were no panels of half a dozen people in those days. We met one on one, the matron and me in her office. I was sixteen, and I had a glowing school reference and reports that positively sang my praises.

"What books do you like to read?" she asked, looking over the brim of her glasses.

"Oh! Shakespeare", I replied, full of enthusiasm.

After all, I had just finished my O'level, and Shakespeare's *Twelfth Night* had been my bedtime reading for the past twelve months. I gushed about the poetry I liked to read and told her that my favourite author was Charles Dickens. I had been reading *David Copperfield* and loved it. I loved all the material I had to read for my O'level English Literature exams. It was all true, but looking back, I don't know what the heck my reading had to do with nursing. The matron must have been impressed, however, because she asked me when could I start work.

"As soon as I finish school. I have a holiday booked, but I can always cancel it", I said. Fool that I was, I couldn't wait to start work.

"No, you must have your holiday first. You can start on August the eighth," she said.

When I told my parents I was going to train to be a nurse, my mother was horrified and tried to talk me out of it. She was the head cook at the North Lonsdale Hospital and had heard one tale too many about parties at the doctors' house. She tried her best to talk me into taking up the teaching course I had also been offered, but after seeing the hospital, I found it quite exciting to think I could be working soon. To persuade her, I said that she would be around to keep an eye on me, and as I was nearly seventeen, it was time I started work.

It was 1966. I had my holiday at Butlin's Holiday Camp and started work a week later than everyone else. Well, one other girl, Liz, also started a week late. As things turned out, Liz and I were to have a lot more in common in the future.

We had already been measured for our uniforms. The ladies in the sewing room all seemed the motherly type and were very nice, but even they dared not hem our dresses as short as we would have liked. As a cadet nurse, my uniform was yellow. My school uniform had been brown and yellow, so there wasn't much difference, apart from the huge cap with an overly large flap that all cadets had to wear. We were given six brand-new uniforms with our names carefully sewn into the neck. The dresses were yellow, the aprons were yellow, and surprisingly, the belts were also yellow. They were not exactly designer dresses. They were boring and practical. Over the next one and a half years, I became an errand girl. I was no longer treated as an adult or given responsibilities. I didn't have a name; I was known as "cadetti". I heard that shouted a hundred times a day.

"Cadetti, can you run down to the store and get me some notes?"

"Cadetti, can you run along to path lab and take these forms?"

I was also known as "Primrose" or "Canary" on account of the colour of the uniform.

There were about two dozen cadets, and we were all known as Primrose, Canary, or Cadetti. I think someone turned the clock back when I wasn't looking; it felt like I was about ten years old again. With the way I was spoken to and the menial tasks I was given to do, it was as if my brain had gone into hibernation.

One of my first placements was in the records office, staffed solely by women, because office work was women's work. One of the office girls was also seventeen; she had peroxide blonde hair that went straight down to her shoulders and then flicked up in a perfect curl. To hold the curl in place, she used so much hairspray. She sort of turned her head, like someone who has a stiff neck, and her hair never moved – it just sort of sat on her head like a helmet. With her perfect make-up – well at least I think it was perfect when I first saw her – I thought she had a couple of spiders sitting on her eyelids, but it was just her starched mascara. With her polished fingernails, she looked older than seventeen. She would be included in the office conversations, where as I was invisible, except when I was needed to go to the record store that just happened to be situated at the farthest point away on the ground floor. It certainly kept me fit – fitter than Mrs Nixon, who was a chain smoker and couldn't complete a sentence without a good old coughing fit. The office was so thick in smoke there were times when I could hardly breathe, let alone Mrs Nixon and all the other 'puffers'.

Then there was a dwarf, Miss Simons. I had never seen a dwarf outside of a circus before and it fascinated me to watch her clamber up onto the chairs. Everything was too big for her. She was probably about four and a half feet tall or maybe a bit less, and there was no special equipment to accommodate her.

Patients coming to casualty had to first register and were given a casualty card. They would tap on a little window that 'Blondie' would 'man', and duly fill out a form. On occasions, Miss Simons would have to answer the window, but by the time she had managed to climb onto the high stool that 'Blondie' perched upon so perfectly like a mannequin, there would inevitably be a more impatient tapping on the window.

"Yes", Miss Simmons would say in a sharp voice as she flung the window open.

Now I know it's not really funny, but she had to kind of stretch over the work top to reach the little window. Bless her; it was such a struggle. She had to kneel on the stool, and try and hold her skirt down at the same time. It was the kind of thing you would see in a comedy film. Watching her try to get off the stool was almost like watching a stunt act. She would slide down, holding the back of the stool 'till her little legs touched the floor, by which time she was quite out of breath and she would huff and puff back to her own chair and sit down with a sigh of relief.

The middle-aged woman in charge of the office made it her priority to make sure no cadet in her office ever had nothing to do. Never would a cadet be allowed to rest outside of her official tea brake. So, while all the office workers could talk to each other, the invisible cadet was given work to do. Things that didn't really need doing but which kept them busy: re-tidying the already tidy shelves – well, as tidy as you can make a stack of patients notes – or worse still, filing the blooming things. Hundreds and hundreds of patients' notes always needed filing. It was all very tiring, mainly because I was on my feet all day when I had been use to sitting down. There were times when I longed to go back behind my school desk, sitting in neat rows, with nothing more to worry about than the next essay to be written or book to be read.

I did get their attention once. At the time, I was doing the Duke of Edinburgh's Gold award scheme – just thought I would drop that in – and I got to go to Buckingham Palace to meet Prince Philip. I had been away on an adventure weekend. One of our activities was archery. It was absolutely brilliant, but what I hadn't noticed was every time I shot an arrow, the string twanged on my arm. We were not given any arm protection quite simply because there wasn't any – only those owned by the members of the archery club, and they were not willing to lend them out. By the time I returned to work on the Monday, my arm sported a very impressive, almost jet black bruise, that started at my wrist and stretched all the way to my elbow, which I must say was a bit on the tender side. It was the first and only time that I was noticed. As all the office staff clucked around me to get a better look, I felt quite important being the centre of attention. It lasted all of five minutes and then it was work as usual.

I did learn how to use a telephone while working in the office, not that I could be trusted to answer one except when I was down in the dungeon, by which I mean the record store, when they would often phone up for extra notes. I had never used a phone before. Not many people had one in their home, and we certainly didn't. The phone had a strange effect on some people. Their voice changed when they picked it up, and they kind of put on a posh accent commonly known as a telephone voice. I don't know if I did that or not, but I suppose I may have done.

The first twelve months passed in a similar environment in various departments around the hospital. Then for the last six months before training started I was allocated a ward. Wow! A taste of real nursing. Hah! I don't think. This was really hard work. I was at everyone's beck and call. One morning, I was called into sister's office. She had been waiting for me to come on duty. A third-year student had reported me for not bagging up the dirty linen the day before. The small fact that no one had told me to bag the dirty linen counted for nothing. I was given a right dressing down. Cadets were at the bottom of the pile when it came to giving out orders and they were the only ones low enough for a student to boss about. Someone needed to knock her off her high and mighty perch but there wasn't much I could do about it.

The ward I was working on was an admission ward, so there were several small rooms, including a nursery. I liked that the best. There were also surgical and medical patients, both male and female. Every day was cleaning day because there was such a high turnover of patients. On another occasion, I was called into sister's office because the domestic had reported that I had dropped a sweet paper on the floor that she had just cleaned. I remember so clearly standing there, being told to apologise, but I swear to God I did not drop that paper. The domestic argued her point that it must have been me, probably for no other reason than that I was the most junior. I was told to go and pick it up. Absolutely no way would I pick up that paper. This was not a good start to my nursing career. It was so unjustified, as no one had ever doubted my word before, but it seemed I had to get use to it. For what seemed an eternity, sister just stared at me without blinking. Then she turned on her heel and said,

"Dismissed".

She stooped down and picked up the wrapper herself. I don't think anyone quite so junior had ever stood up to a sister before. My friends said I should have picked it up anyway, but it was just the injustice of the situation that prevented me from doing so. The next morning, the domestic brought in a home-made trifle. She was always toadying up to sister, but on this occasion, she came looking for me.

"Come and get some trifle, cadet", she said, with a grin on her face.

That was her way of apologising. I nearly told her where to shove it, but she made a pretty mean trifle so I tucked in.

My only experience of life had been school, so to me this seemed an extremely harsh regime. Working in a hospital was very hard work with very little praise. Except for the patients, who treated you with total respect and followed to the letter any instructions given to them. Sometimes the higher ranking did have a sense of humour, albeit a bit warped. I had been warned about the tricks played on April Fool's Day, and I must say I was dreading any forthcoming embarrassment; I blushed so easily. So it came as quite a relief when sister casually said to me,

"Cadet, go to pharmacy and get a Bowman's Capsule".

I was relieved because having passed my O'Level human biology I knew instantly that the Bowman's Capsule was a part in the kidneys. I allowed myself a small smile and I opened my mouth to say something like, "April Fool", but sister was quicker, and having gone to a lot of trouble to arrange a neatly packaged April Fool bag that the boss in pharmacy had to hand to me, she was determined to carry it through.

"Go along cadet. Don't just stand there", she said with a straight face.

I snuck along to the kitchens to ask my mother what should I do.

"You will just have to go along with it", she said.

I even asked the lady in the pharmacy. She was apologetic and said Sister O'Donnell played the same trick every year. There was another cadet who was sent to C.S.S.D. (central sterilising supply unit), for a purse string suture. Although there is such a thing, it is a procedure, not a special thread as she had been told. I took the empty bag labelled Bowman's Capsule back to the ward and opened it as instructed to find a piece of paper saying April Fool. Sister thought it was hilarious and tittered away to herself. At leased it put her in a good mood for the rest of the day. I could just imagine what it was like in the sister's sitting room as they all told each other about their April Fool's tricks.

Anyway, the good thing was that I was in a hospital environment and I was a working girl, not a schoolgirl, and the wages came in handy. I made some good friends. One in particular, called Claire, whenever we went out, she attracted attention because she had a laugh like a hyena. Her high-pitched screech could be heard above the loudest din. You should have heard her when 'Ob-La-Di, Ob-La-Da' by the Marmalade came on the juke box. She would shriek,

"Ooo, it"s my song",

and go into peels of laughter that could be heard all over the pub.

During the time I spent cadetting, I didn't think I was learning anything, but surprisingly I learnt an awful lot, which stood me in good stead later on – including protocol. The first time I had used the dining room, I finished my meal and was going to dash along to tell my mother, who was at work in the kitchens, all about my first day. I got up to leave. Big mistake! How was I to know you had to leave in strict rotation of seniority? Higher than me was, well, everyone, except other cadets. Sisters generally ate at a different time to other nursing staff, but if any were in the dining room they left first, followed by the staff nurses, the enrolled nurses (E.N.), the students, and finally the cadets. If there was a slow eater or someone who was busy talking, we all just sat there, waiting for them to finish. Only nursing staff were allowed to use this dining room. Ancillary staff, domestics, and porters all ate in a different dining room. You were not encouraged to mix. I was called to the front of the room to where the assistant matron was sitting. She would have made a good ventriloquist because she hissed through lips that barely moved.

"Sit down, cadet, and wait your turn before leaving", she instructed.

With my cheeks burning a bright crimson, I went meekly back to my seat. My turn to leave came when the room was nearly empty and there were just the cadets left.

Working as a cadet gave an insight into what it would be like to work in a hospital. It was during this time that some cadets left, realising that nursing was not for them. Or they wanted more money, and they would leave to work in a factory or somewhere paying better wages, which was just about everywhere.

The hospital was an old Victorian building that had been built with donations from the local public, who paid something like a penny a week to use it. Barrow-in-Furness had developed around heavy industries, such as iron ore mines, steelworks, and shipbuilding. There was plenty of work for the hospital. They say that in 1949, the year after the National Health Service was introduced, the number of people using casualty doubled from the previous year. This was also the year I was born.

Along with the health service came a whole range of immunisation programmes for children. My mother thought there were far too many injections for a young child, so she refused to let me have some of them. I just had the injections that she thought was necessary. It was great at the time. I didn't have all the needles the other kids had, but when I started at the hospital, I had to have all the injections I had missed: polio, smallpox, and whatever else I had missed out on.

We worked a forty-hour week and were paid the princely sum of £270 per year, about five pounds a week, that went down to four pounds ten shillings when we reached eighteen, on account of having to pay into a pension fund. The excitement of picking up my first pay packet is still clear in my mind. I can remember standing in the pay queue and being handed the small brown pay envelope with real cash inside. I felt rich. I had to give exactly half of my wages to my mam for my keep. There wasn't enough left to go out and paint the town red, but it was more than my pocket money, and right from that first pay day I saved a little bit for a rainy day.

As cadets we went to the local collage on a two-day release scheme to study human biology, and French or English for the ones who didn't already have an O'level. We worked a five and a half day week, finishing at twelve O"clock Saturday dinnertime for the weekend. It took a bit of getting used to, working full time. It was tiring running backward and forward all day. I was glad the uniform had included those sensible lace-up shoes, but if we thought this was hard, it was nothing compared to what was to come.

CHAPTER TWO

I could hardly contain my excitement when the day came that I was to go into preliminary training school, known as P.T.S. I had long since got over my disappointment of not working with animals. I guess humans were the next best thing.

My excitement was tinged with sadness because Claire had not been accepted to do the State Registration Training. She had to do the Enrolled Nurse Training, which was based in the Geriatric hospital a couple of miles down the road. She was such a gentle, caring person I could never understand this decision, even though the reason was she didn't have enough O'levels. Matron could have used her discretion if she wanted to, but it was not to be. She did stay in the same nurses' home, however, so we saw plenty of each other.

It was compulsory for all student nurses to live in at the nurses' home for at least the first twelve months of training. In fact, they are normally residents for two years except by special arrangement. It seemed all the buildings around the hospital had been bought up for hospital employees. There were two nurses' homes, on Church Street and Albert Street. They had previously been rows of terraced houses that had been knocked through to make a maze of assorted rooms. There was a doctors' house and several of the houses from surrounding streets had been converted into flats for the married doctors.

We had been given a list of things we had to bring with us. These included black shoes and stockings – at least three pairs of stockings, and our shoes had to be the "good, lace-up variety, with rubber, not plastic, heels".

There was a whole group of us moving in at the same time. We had all been to the linen room to collect clean linen for our beds, and then we had been told to wait in the sitting room for the home sister. When she arrived, we were instructed to follow her, like little ducklings following their mother, as she allocated a room to each of us. I was so excited. I had never been away from home before. Mind you, I only lived a mile down the road, and with my mother also working at the hospital, it was hardly likely that I would get homesick.

When my turn came to be shown my room, the door was pushed open and immediately bounced shut again. I narrowly missed getting a busted nose. I tried again by gently leaning against it, and then I peered around the door. I thought there had been a mistake; surely this must be the broom cupboard. The door wouldn't open fully because the bed was behind it. It was the smallest bed I had ever seen. I remember thinking that it must have been made for a pigmy, and I felt certain I wouldn't fit into it. There was also a wardrobe that I could just about squeeze past, a chest of drawers, and a sink in the corner. I could stand in the middle of the room and touch the walls on either side. No kidding, it was a good job I didn't suffer from claustrophobia, and just to make matters worse, the tiny window overlooked the morgue. I soon learnt that I would be woken on a regular basis through the night by the sounds of a trolley being taken over the yard with a body on it. All the larger rooms were kept for the overseas nurses. We were instructed that visitors may be asked into the home, but students were to notify the home sister if they wished to invite anyone in, and communal sitting rooms to be vacated by eleven P.M.

After we had made up our beds, we were all to meet in the sitting room to introduce ourselves. Most of us had been cadets and we knew each other, but there were some outsiders. I braced myself for what

I knew was to come. I had been secretly hoping that one of the new girls would have a name that could be made fun of, but no, everyone else had said their name and they were all run-of-the-mill type names and now it was my turn.

"My name is Beryl", I said quietly.

"What did you say", someone said. "Speak up".

"My name is Beryl", I said a little louder.

The reaction was instant. "O! The peril. It's Beryl the peril".

And then everyone collapsed into laughter. I had heard it a million times before. I curse the person whoever penned the name of "Beryl the peril", because I have never lived it down. The stigma of that name follows me everywhere. I suppose after one and a half years of only my friends knowing my name, I had to get it over with sometime that my name wasn't really Brenda or Tracey or whatever other name I had called myself.

Of course "Beryl the peril" was a comic strip character that came out in the "50s. At least I hope it was the '50s, 'cause if it was any earlier that means I would have already been born, and my parents would have had a lot to answer for. Beryl, in the comic, was always getting into trouble. She was on a par with Dennis the Menace and Minnie the Minx. I blame my name for the fact that I did seem to get into more than my fair share of trouble. I had learnt long ago not to get mad, but to get even, which was how June, who after repeatedly being told I did not like her name-calling, became June the balloon, on account of her being quite stout. She had been tormenting me mercilessly over the weekend, and when I went into work on the Monday I was greeted with,

"O! It's the peril".

"O! It's June the balloon", I replied.

Heaven only knows why after all the stick she had given me, but she was mortified and kept asking me was she really like a balloon.

"Yes", I told her unsympathetically.

She didn't like her new name but she never again called me 'the peril'.

I went to bed early on my first night, in my tiny bed, wondering what P.T.S. would be like. I didn't get much sleep because every time I turned over I fell onto the floor. It seemed like I had just nodded off, when I heard an almighty banging on the door next to mine. I nearly fell out of bed again. "Bloody 'ell', I thought. "What is going on?" Then I heard it repeated again and again, accompanied by a loud,

"Wake up, nurse. It's six thirty".

"Blimey!" I thought. At the very least the place must be on fire, but no, it was the night sister waking up the early shift. The only problem was, of course, everyone else got woken at the same time.

There was no point in trying to go back to sleep now, so I got washed and dressed and went over to the dining room for breakfast. The assistant matron sat at the head of the room. Her face looked like a bulldog chewing a wasp. Her long grey hair was pulled tightly back into a bun, and not a single strand escaped. The creation was topped off with a rather cute little lace-trimmed cap perched right on the top of her head. She could turn a grown man into a quivering jelly with just one look, and you never, ever answered her back.

The point of her being there at this time was to make sure we all ate our breakfast. I could hardly believe it when I first learnt we had to eat our food, or at least try a little of everything. It seems that because the 'coming of age' was twenty-one, the sister was in loco parentis because we were only eighteen. That meant the sister was like a surrogate mother. Yuk! Her 'job' was to make sure we ate our food. Breakfast, for me, was not to big a problem, but when it came to dinner and certain vegetables, that's another story. It's strange to think I am now a vegetarian and that I practically live off vegetables. I had always been a picky eater, and this was to bring me to sisters' attention on many occasions.

After breakfast, I made my way to the classroom, loaded up with the books we had been told to buy. It was a small room in the nurses' home. The school of nursing had just taken over an empty bank that was over the road, and it was being converted into a new classroom and practical room, but it wouldn"t be ready until the following year.

Some of the others were already there. We were to spend every day of the next six weeks in this classroom. We had already been issued uniforms that were a lovely lilac colour. The length of our dresses had been determined by our kneeling down; the hem had to touch the floor, so that it covered our knees. After all, this was the swinging '60s – the age of the mini skirt and all that. At last I was out of that awful yellow dress, but the stiff, white dog collar held in place with a metal stud felt like it was choking me. It had a mind of it's own, and on a regular basis pinged open. We didn't have to wear that unless we went on a ward. I had tied my long, dark hair into a neat pony tail before going over for breakfast, but it seems it wasn't neat enough, as it was touching my collar. I knew it shouldn't have, but I thought that since I was in the classroom it would be okay.

"Start out as we mean to go on, nurse", I was told sternly.

I was sent away to tidy myself up. My hair had to be pinned up underneath. I was not the only one; there were several of us, so I didn"t feel too bad.

When we returned, we had to have our nails inspected. We had to hold our hands up, and if our nails showed above the fingertip, they were for the chop – the nails, that is, not our fingers. After that, all trace of nail varnish had to be removed. Those of us who had been cadets knew all these basic rules, so we were better prepared. We were allowed some make-up, but only sparingly. I never wore it at work, so that didn't affect me. Finally, only nursing studs were allowed as earrings, and definitely no jewellery except a wedding ring. The uniform was finished off with black lace-up shoes and black tights. We didn't wear the starched aprons or belts until we went on the wards, and the whole lot was completed with a cloak – not the brown one with the green lining we had worn as cadets, but a proper nurses one. The cloaks were all colour coded – navy blue on the outside, with a pale blue lining for sister, a red lining for a staff nurse, and students, and enrolled nurses, known as pupils during training, wore green. The cloaks had long ties that crossed over at the front and fastened behind your back. The cloak was a symbol of being a real nurse. Nurses had worn cloaks ever since the days of Florence Nightingale. They came in very useful on cold nights. Wrapped tightly around your body, they were lovely and warm.

The worst was yet to come. For the folding of the cap, you needed a degree in origami. We were given a shaped piece of starched material that had to be folded meticulously into something that perched precariously on your head like an ornament. Being a cadet had come in useful after all. We already knew how to fold caps, but the new girls didn't have a clue.

As first-year student nurses, our caps had one red line on them. Second years had two red lines, and third years had three. When you finally made the grade and passed your exams, a thick red stripe denoted that you were a staff nurse, but that was a heck of a long way into the future for me. Those caps caused so many problems over the years. They were either blown off, knocked off, or fell off of their own accord. It was only the female nurses who had to wear them. There were not many male nurses, but the one or two who did exist didn't wear caps, as the caps didn't serve any useful purpose except as a target for any passing porter to flick off. I thought that was rather sexist. Caps were a relic from the Victorian days, when the nurses' heads had to be completely covered to prevent the spread of nits.

Nurse training in the '60s was based on the apprenticeship model, with most of our knowledge being learnt while working on the wards. Throughout the six weeks of P.T.S., we were taught all the basics of what made a good nurse. We were taught how to administer bed baths, how to make beds with sharp, hospital corners, and how to drag lift a patient up the bed. What was that? Drag lift? Yes, that's right. We were taught to drag lift patients. No wonder so many of us ended up with back problems. We practiced giving injections by sticking needles into an orange. We used glass syringes, and several of them got broken as our shaky hands dropped them on the floor, where they smashed into smithereens. Nothing was thrown away; everything was sent for sterilising and reused. Sometimes the plungers on the syringes would stick when they hadn't been dried properly before packing. They would suddenly brake free and go flying across the room. We were also taught how to give all around general care.

From time to time we would be taken to a ward to put into practise what we had learnt in the classroom. When we went to give our first injections, we were suppose to give an air of confidence as we approached the patient. My hands were trembling so much it's a wonder the needle found the target. I was going over the instructions in my head: mentally divide the buttocks into quarters and aim for the upper, outer quadrangle. Boy, was I glad when that was over. I often wondered what went through the patients' minds when they saw a group of trainees arriving on the ward. You could almost hear them thinking, like something out of the "Carry On" films, "Cor, blimey, it's time for target practise again".

The wards were Nightingale style. That meant that there was one large room with beds down both sides, about thirty all together on the surgical wards, and a few less on the medical side. At the bottom of the ward were large windows that were opened every day to let fresh air blow through. When the ward was full and there was no more bed space, another line of beds was put down the middle, which made it very difficult to manoeuvre trolleys or anything else about the ward, and there was no privacy for the patients. It didn't take long to learn that what we practised in the classroom could not always be carried out on a busy main ward.

We soon settled into a routine, and the days passed quickly. There was so much to learn. At the end of P.T.S., we had our exams to sit. The nurse who came top was awarded the P.T.S. prize. When the results were given out, I had come top. I was so excited until the announcement was quickly followed with a statement:

"Nurse Park, you were given instructions to write the answer to each question on a new sheet of paper, but as you wrote yours on a new side of paper. I have deducted four percent, which puts you in second place".

Well! Was there need for that over-the-top punishment? I thought that it was way below the belt. Talk about feeling cheated, I was gutted, but the decision was final and I just had to accept it, though that didn't stop me from grumbling. I thought it most unfair.

At this point, we were given the rest of our uniforms, including six very starched aprons that were so stiff they stood up on their own. The bibs or top of the aprons were held in place by two safety pins, but with all that starch it was quite difficult to push the pin through without bending it or sticking it through your finger. We were also issued three very starched belts and three very starched collars that were held in place with a collar stud that felt like it was choking you, as it stuck into your Adams Apple, but for all that, I must say they did look ever so neat and tidy. I felt I looked the part of a proper nurse.

There was one more thing I had to endure before formally starting work on the wards. I can honestly say it was the most embarrassing moment of my life – the obligatory medical. Now you have to remember that this was in the days when you only spoke to your immediate superior. It was only on rare occasions that you spoke to anyone more than one level above yourself, and I had gone to an all-girls school, and was very modest about anyone seeing my body. We also had a particularly strict headmistress, who would walk briskly into morning assembly with the familiar black cloak forming a trail behind her, the mortar-board that was oh, so tempting to knock off her head, and proceed to lecture us on the virtues of not looking into the boys playground, which we had to pass to get to the canteen. I thought we would be struck blind or something equally bad if we dared to look at a boy, let alone talk to one. They were an alien species that had to be avoided at all costs. Did I mention she was a spinster? Well, she was. No surprise there then.

So, when I was sent to the medical clinic to be seen by a consultant, it was nerve racking to say the least. Upon arrival, I was told to take all my clothes off, everything apart from my knickers. Obviously, no one here had heard of preserving modesty. No gowns were available, but there again, they weren't available for any patients either. It just wasn't thought necessary. I was told to lie on a couch, and was covered with a blanket, which I held tightly right up to my chin. The medicals were carried out when all other clinics had finished, so it was deadly quiet. Then, in the distance I could hear the sound of footsteps; it sounded like an army was approaching. The door was flung open and in marched the consultant and a sister. Without saying a single word, and with one swift movement, he pulled the blanket off me and threw it on the floor. He nearly pulled my bloody nails out, I'd been holding on so tight. My face had turned a deep crimson colour. And what did I say? Well, nothing of relevance. I sort of stammered,

"My feet are black because I had new shoes on and the dye has come out".

"Really", he said with a huge smirk on his face.

I hadn't been this embarrassed since I first had to wear my gym knickers in public. When I was at school, I can remember cringing behind the curtain on the side of the stage when I first put on the bloomers that I had made in the needlework class. At school, we had to make our own gym kit, which consisted of the olive green knickers, a leaf-green blouse that was more like a parachute with elastic round the bottom, and a skirt that didn't get made until our third year. It all had to be made big enough to last until we left school. The heavy material and the colour were relicts from the Second World War, when material was in short supply. All other schools had changed to shorts, and the colour of their uniforms long ago, but not the 'Alfs'. The knickers were one size fits all. We had to sew up the sides and put elastic round the waist and each leg. They were definitely like granny bloomers, and the blouses were not much better, with elastic round the bottom. Every time you stretched up, the blouse shot up your chest, and as I played shooter in netball, I had to hang onto the bottom of it with one hand while positioning the ball in the other hand, constantly pulling it down, to remain modest. It wasn't to bad for the first couple of years, but then I guess I just out grew it.

Right then, I would have given my right arm to have that curtain to hide behind, or the parachute of a blouse. This consultant seemed to enjoy my embarrassment as I squirmed while he examined me. I was glad when it was finally over, but that was not the end of it. I was sent for a chest x-ray; we had to have a chest x-ray every year. Once again, I had to take my uniform off. Well, at least lower it down to my waist, which I think was more embarrassing than removing it, as all my pens, pencil, and scissors fell out of the pockets. I left them all on the floor; I wasn't going to bend down with bare boobs. I remember thinking, "Could this day get any worse?" as I was positioned against a cold metal plate. A young male radiographer carried out my x-ray. I can't think of anything more excruciatingly embarrassing. I was glad when the whole thing was over, but to give him his due, he seemed as embarrassed as me.

We were all allocated to a ward, in general the male surgical ward, which was coupled with Orthopaedics, and was the busiest in the hospital, but we found that the men did try and help themselves, whereas the women made the most of a rest and expected everything to be done for them. Female wards were nicknamed bedpan alley, because you couldn't walk down the ward without someone asking for a bedpan, and once one person asked, it set off a chain reaction and half the ward would want one.

CHAPTER THREE

Running along side the working life of a student nurse was the social life of teenage girls who just happened to be student nurses. We were never short of attention. When asked,

"What work do you do?" we'd reply,

"I'm a student nurse',

Although it could get a bit boring when you heard for the hundredth time,

"Will you show me the kiss of life?" or, "How about giving me a bed bath?"

But try explaining that even though you were eighteen years old, you had to be back in the nurses" home by ten thirty or you were in big trouble. It was usually met with disbelief. I can't blame them. When I first discovered this little gem, I didn't believe it either. It was with total shock and horror that I discovered that the doors to the nurses' home were all locked at 10:30 P.M. After that, if you were late in, you had to go to the night sisters office for the keys and a lecture on the importance of a good night's sleep. You were allowed one late pass per week until 11:00 P.M., but if you were late more than once in the same week, you were on report and had to go to the matron's office. I was to get into trouble so many times in the year to come just for getting back late. To start with, at least, everyone was in on time. No one wanted to give a bad impression.

The working week had just been reduced to a forty-hour week from a forty-two-hour week. As students, we had to work shifts, but not the split shifts that the trained nurses worked; they were awful. You had to work four hours, go home for four hours, and then return to work for another four hours. Working shifts was hard enough to get use to. It wasn't the week on 'earlies', or a week on 'lates' that factory workers worked, but usually you worked until nine at night and then returned at seven in the morning. Suddenly, there was no routine to your day. You'd eat dinner at three o'clock one day and twelve o'clock the next. It played havoc with your constitution.

When I first stepped onto a ward in uniform, it was so daunting. I gazed down rows of beds, knowing that patients were going to ask questions that I probably didn't know the answers to, and ask me to do things for them – maybe personal things – that could be embarrassing, but I had to be confident. That was the answer to everything.

At the start of each shift, we went into the sisters' office for the handover. This was when we were brought up to date on new admissions, treatments, and anything of relevance. I felt like a fish out of water. Everyone looked very knowledgeable, where as I couldn't even pronounce half the words, let alone know what they meant. The sister or the nurse in charge would read off a list of patients' names and their treatments, so you might hear, 'A Mr T. Brown had a Vagotomy and Pyloroplasty yesterday, and he is on hourly fluids of one ounce of water', or, 'Mr B. Smith has had a Cholecystectomy. He is allowed out of bed today'. Blimey, it sounded like she had swallowed a dictionary. Things did get clearer once we learnt that there was a pattern to the words, such as anything ending in 'otomy' meant to open into, or if it ended in 'it is' it meant inflammation, while anything ending in 'ectomy' meant removal of. There were lots of these little gems, and once we had learnt them life became a bit easier.

Ward routines were continuous rounds of one kind or another: cleaning rounds, matron's rounds, doctor's rounds, dressing rounds, bedpan rounds, drinks rounds, back rounds, blood-pressure rounds, and the adding up of the fluid balance charts. There were so many rounds I felt dizzy. The sister or nurse in charge would make out a work rota at the start of the shift. Everyone was allocated different jobs, and if you got finished first, you then helped out the others. Everyone knew exactly what they were doing, and the sister knew exactly who to go to if a job wasn't done. The first-year students obviously got the most menial tasks, but gradually they would be teamed up with someone more senior to do the more skilled work.

Starting with the cleaning, there was basic cleaning to be done every day, but once a week, all the beds were pulled into the middle of the ward so that the domestic could clean the floor properly. Everything was washed, starting with the curtain rails, the beds, and the lockers. Every day, a fresh paper bag was stuck to the side of the lockers for the patients to put their rubbish in. You name it, and it was washed. The curtains were changed every month, and everyone helped with the cleaning. Where was the poor, old, first-year student? Why, in the sluice, of course, where she spent most of her life! The sluice was considered a worse job than general cleaning, except by the nurses who smoked, because they often had a sneaky drag while cleaning up when they were sent down there. Although the bedpans were washed in a washer, they also had to be polished and dried, along with urine bottles, vomit bowls, sputum dishes, and denture mugs. Everything was made of stainless steel, and everything had to be polished 'till you could see your face in them. Not that I wanted to look any longer than necessary into the bottom of these essentials, but you get the picture.

Anyone who ever went to a hospital commented on the smell, and anyone who worked there seemed to have the permanent smell of disinfectant. It was, of course, Sudol. No germs could survive the onslaught of the liberal use of Sudol.

The dressing rounds followed strict procedures as well. At least half an hour before the round started, all the curtains were drawn around the beds to allow for any dust to settle. There were always two nurses to do the dressings, a 'dirty' nurse and a 'sterile' nurse. During this time, patients were confined to bed. No one was allowed to sit on the beds. They either had to be in them, or sit in a chair, but they definitely could not sit on the bed. The male patients had to have a full set of pyjamas on. No bare chests were allowed. The ward doors would be closed, and walking up and down the ward was kept to a minimum while dressings were carried out. It would have to be an emergency before anyone was allowed onto the ward, and that included the doctors.

One thing every student had to do as soon as possible was to lay out a body, which was never an easy thing to do. This wasn't quite my first encounter with a dead body. During P.T.S., we were sent over to watch a post mortem. We entered the room to find that the PM was under way. There was this human being cut open like a side of beef at the butcher's shop, with his scalp peeled back to expose his brain, and his chest slit open to reveal his heart and lungs. There should have been a revolving door on that room, because I was out of there so fast my feet hardly touched the ground. This was the same man we had seen the day before in the intensive care unit. There were so many things wrong with him, including multiple organ failures, that I did wonder why it was necessary to inflict this last piece of indignity on him.

The body in front of me now had to be given a full wash, have his dentures put in place, and then be dressed in a cotton shroud. To this day, I still can't wear a blouse with ruffles around the neck, wrists, or down the front because that was how the shrouds were made. After washing and dressing the body, it then had to be wrapped in a sheet that went underneath first and then over the front, to be elaborately folded over the head and feet until the person looked like a mummy. It was at this point that I got a fit of the giggles. As we turned him over to place the sheet under him, the shock of holding a dead weight, no pun intended, took me by surprise, and he nearly went straight onto the floor. Then the arms and legs took on a life of their own as they flopped over the side of the bed. I struggled to keep him from falling off. Then there was the revulsion I felt at having to handle a dead body so close to me. I felt so guilty giggling at a time like this, but it was made worse by the fact that we knew that other patients could hear us, and trying to stifle the giggles with the pretence of a cough only made matters worse. This was the precise time that I suddenly realised I needed the loo. So, there I was, cross-legged, stifling a laugh, and struggling to keep a large corpse from crashing onto the floor.

The job was finally finished, with the feet being tied together with a bandage to hold them in place. A name tag had been tied onto the big toe, and a second pinned to the chest that would be used to put on the front of the drawer of the fridge where he would be taken. After what seemed an eternity, the body was almost ready to be taken over to the morgue. The final thing to do was to find a couple of flowers. No one was ever taken to the morgue without a small posy of flowers placed on the chest. This initiation into the handling of a dead body didn't quite finish with the removal of the body. When the porter arrived with the not-very-discreet trolley covered with a purple and gold velvet cloth, there would usually be a second porter waiting over at the morgue, especially if it was dark, as the morgue was outside and across the yard. The poor student would be breathing a sigh of relief that her first laying out was over, and then she would be instructed to pull out a fridge drawer in order to put the body in, and a porter covered in a sheet would be waiting to scare the life out of her. Many a nurse ran screaming across the yard looking as white as a ghost. I didn't think this would happen to me, because having been a cadet, I knew all about the porters' silly little trick. So why did I nearly jump out of my skin when the lights suddenly went out and I realised that the porter had disappeared?

"You're not funny", I shouted out nervously. "I know you're there".

There was still not a sound. Then, like a bolt out of the blue, I was grabbed from behind. My God! I nearly had a heart attack, not to mention wet my knickers.

"You bloody idiot", I shouted. "You nearly gave me a heart attack".

The porter thought it was hilarious, and he laughed his socks off. When I got back to the ward, I was sent to get a cup of tea 'in order to collect myself together'. We were always allowed time for a cup of tea after the first laying out.

The working days were long and very hard work, but in general, once the initial nerves wore off, it was enjoyable, and we soon settled down into the ward routines. We enjoyed ourselves socially, and we didn't need a lot of money, which was just as well. We actually got thirteen pounds a month after our board had been deducted, so we couldn't exactly go on a mad spending spree. The hospital being in the town meant that we did not have to use transport, and when we did go out, we could make half a lager last all night if necessary.

One night while in a town centre bar called the Dreadnaught, which was in the Majestic Hotel – this was before the days of our small town getting any nightclubs – there was a group of four young lads drinking their pints of beer. One of them had previously been a patient on the orthopaedic ward, and my friend Dianne had nursed him.

"Let's go over", she said. "I'll ask him how he's doing".

I quite liked the look of his friend, and as there were four of us, it seemed a good idea, so we agreed, and over we went and casually struck up a conversation. John, who had had a fractured leg, was getting along fine.

"What's your friend's name?" Dianne asked.

"Ray", he replied. "And your friend is?"

"Beryl".

Never backward in coming forward, Dianne said, "Beryl, this is Ray. Ray, this is Beryl".

So Ray and I were left talking. He seemed a bit shy. He was tall and lanky, with curly hair. Having a conversation with him was like pulling hens' teeth. I discovered that he was an apprentice joiner, and that he was nineteen. He seemed very nice, but at the end of the night he just said, "Goodnight", and went off without asking to see me again. We all made our way back to the nurses' home not expecting to see him again.

There were times when 'living in' felt a bit like being a prisoner. We knew that blocks had been put on all the downstairs sash windows so that they only opened about six inches, which was designed to protect us from intruders, but if ever there had been a fire, I shudder to think what might have happened. One window had been forgotten, and as the months passed and we got a little more daring, we would arrange for a friend to unlock the window if we thought we might be late back in. There was often a steady stream of nurses waiting to get a 'bunk up' from their boyfriends to climb through the open window.

One night, waiting as usual, we discovered that blocks had been put on that day and we were locked out. Some rat had snitched to the home sister, and without warning they had been put on immediately. That meant someone had to be brave enough to go to the sister's office and ask for the key. Why did it always have to be me? I could answer that myself. Because I tend to be a bit mouthy, I suppose I was considered brave. Brave or foolish I don't know, but I sneaked up the back stairs. One advantage of the old building was having a back flight of stairs that ran directly from the kitchens to the dinning room. Night sisters' office was just down the corridor. I hovered around at the top until I saw the night sister leave to do her rounds and then I dashed in, grabbed the keys, and ran as fast as I could back to the others.

I unlocked the door at the end of the tunnel that connected the nurses' home to the hospital, and one nurse waited to keep the door open for me while I ran back with the keys. The night sister was still out, and I managed to replace the keys without her ever knowing they had gone.

I went straight up to my room and got ready for bed, but as I tried to get into bed, my legs couldn't go down. Something was stopping them. This was my first taste of an 'apple pie bed'. While I had returned the keys, my mates had quickly remade my bed by doubling up the lower sheet so that it only went down half way. While I was still trying to work out what was happening, the door burst open and three heads appeared round the door. My mates, giggling like mad, shouted,

"Surprise! Do you like your bed?"

Well, no, I didn't, actually. It was late at night, I was tired, and now I had to start and make my bed again.

"No, I flipping well don't", I replied. "The next time you want a mug to go and get the keys you can go yourself", I said grumpily.

Sensing that I wasn't best pleased, they all beat a hasty retreat.

On another night, after going into town and after drinking two or three halves of lager, Liz and

I decided that we would not be told what time we had to be in. We were eighteen going on nineteen, after all, not babies, so we stayed out late. When we got back to the nurses' home, our courage abruptly left us. Neither one of us would go and ask for the keys. We had no choice but to walk all the way to Liz's house, the best part of a mile. By then, it was eleven thirty. The next morning, we had to get up at about 5:30 A.M., walk back to the nurses' home, and wait for the night sister to open up. As the sister went up one flight of stairs, we ran up the back stairs and jumped into bed fully dressed and pretended to be asleep. When she put her head round the door to make sure we were awake, ready for our early shift, we each tried to sound suitably sleepy.

The first year passed in a blur of work, school, and socialising. We would go into town once or twice a week. It was hardly one long round of parties. We didn't have two halfpennies to rub together, and any boys we met were usually apprentices, so they didn't have much money either. I had met up with Ray again; we seemed to hit it off. He was serving a five-year apprenticeship. He had to learn a bit about all other building trades as well as his own. After a few weeks, we started to go steady.

As time passed, we all gained in confidence and experience as we were rotated to different wards. It wasn't all happy. There were many times when we would gather in one of the rooms and talk for hours, listening to each other's problems, comforting the ones who got upset over being on the sharp end of a sister's tongue, or when a patient they had become close to died. I suppose these days it would be called counselling, but in those days we had each other. We also had the hospital's men of cloth – the priest or vicar who never asked your religion. They not only visited the patients, but they were excellent listeners for the staff as well.

North Lonsdale was an acute patient hospital, and quite small, but it catered for all medical and surgical routines and emergencies. Then there were several satellite hospitals. There was a children's hospital at Devonshire Road, and on the same site an isolation unit and a medical/geriatric ward that originally had been built for T.B. patients. Built on the top of a hill, it had a panoramic view of the local cemetery, complete with crematorium. Was it built so close for any particular reason, or was it just a coincidence that the next-door neighbours all happened to be six feet under? It wouldn"t exactly inspire confidence for the T.B. patients.

On the nice days, we would take a variety of old, battered prams and pushchairs, pile the children in, and go for a walk in the cemetery for some fresh air. The children didn't realise where they were walk-ing, of course, but I did wonder what the adults on the isolation unit and the long-stay medical ward thought as they looked out of the windows and saw a group of nurses and children walking among the gravestones.

Then, of course, there was a separate maternity hospital, called Risedale, and a separate burns unit that also use to have a T.B ward. This was based at High Carley at Ulverston. All these hospitals have since been razed to the ground and housing estates built on the sites.

The gynaecological and geriatric hospital was based in the old workhouse at Roose. It wouldn't be very PC to call it geriatric these days; it would be care of the elderly. Some of the patients on these wards had been there since their teens for such 'crimes' as having a baby outside of marriage, or in the case of one man, he had developed syphilis as a teenager that was said to have sent him blind and mad. He sat all day from morning 'till night saying,

"Poor little blind boy. Poor little blind boy".

Although the hospital was based in lovely grounds, there was no getting away from the dark, austere building towering on the top of a hill, over-looking the town on one side and the gas storage tanks and the shipyard at the back, and open fields to the front. If you went to the top floor, there was an uninterrupted view of the sea. There was a field alongside the hospital that was used by the workhouse inmates to grow their own food. It was not called the workhouse for nothing. They had to work hard growing food and taking in laundry to pay for their keep.

The first thing you noticed when you entered the hospital was the stench of urine. It was quite overpowering. The wards were smaller than the town hospital. They had been divided into two, half for sleeping and half as a sitting area. The patients just sat there all day, staring into space. They could walk around the grounds if they wanted, but not many did. Things were gradually and very slowly starting to change, with physiotherapists going in once or twice a week to try and encourage some of them to move. The trouble was, it was voluntary, and not many volunteered.

One man, Fred, had been there from his early teens, and he was then in his eighties. He would walk to the town hospital, about one and a half miles away, with messages. When he walked, he was like a man on a mission. He never spoke to anyone, never looked right or left, except, I presume, when he crossed the one road that took him to the other hospital, not that there were many cars around. He would deliver his written message to the matron and then walk straight back again. Another man, Walter, would clean the matron's car every week.

It was at this hospital that the story first emerged of the student nurse who was asked to clean all the patients' false teeth. She got a large bowl and collected them all together, soaked them, and gave them all a good scrub. They came up really well. She was feeling quite pleased with herself until she realised, too late, that she had no idea how to identify which dentures belonged to which patient. Oh, boy, did sparks fly! The sister was not best pleased. Most of the patients didn't know their own names, but when it came to the comfort of their own teeth, that was a different matter. It took several days to sort those teeth out. I swear that that student wasn't me, and I promise, Shirley, that I won't tell anyone your real name.

I didn't like working here. The people here weren't ill, but they no longer knew how to look after themselves. They had become institutionalised. They were sad, they were lonely, and they no longer knew how to do anything for themselves, as they were so use to being told what to do, and having everything done for them, from cooking to washing to cleaning. There was nothing for them to even think about. Without their routine they were totally lost. This place epitomised all the reasons why so many old folk were scared stiff of going into a home. It is nothing like that these days, not least because it's been knocked down, but from the very fact that a former workhouse was used to look after the elderly, it was understandable where their fears came from.

I don't think anyone had ever left the workhouse to live elsewhere for decades, not even after it was taken over as a hospital in 1948. Most of the old folk who lived in the town could never forget the stigma attached to the history of what the workhouse stood for, and they would look upon being sent there with terror. You could always tell a workhouse because they were nearly always built on a hill towering over the town, and were always big, imposing buildings. The Roose workhouse was built of sandstone. I don't know how thick the walls were, but the local houses that were built of sandstone had walls between one and a half to two feet thick, so I guess that these were even thicker. I often wonder what kind of a person dreamt up such draconian measures for the poor.

When the government of the day passed a bill called 'Care in the Community', gradually places were found in residential homes for these poor people whom life had passed by, until the Roose former workhouse of Barrow-in-Furness was finally closed down many years later, and finally demolished in the nineteen nineties.

Of course, there were all kinds of tales of ghosts walking the upper floors – the tormented souls of people long since departed. Every hospital had a ghost, usually a lady in grey, but Roose was different because the ghost there was of a young unmarried girl. In the late Victorian days, a young lass called Jenny Stevens became pregnant outside of marriage, and her parents disowned her. To be pregnant and unmarried was a sin. She was put in the workhouse, 'to mend her wicked ways'.

She was just sixteen years old when her baby was born on a freezing cold night in the middle of winter. She wasn't allowed to see it, because it would be sent for adoption to a 'decent, God-fearing family'. They told her it was for the best. She heard her baby crying that night and followed the sounds along the corridor until she found it, a baby boy. They had never told her if it was a boy or a girl. She picked him up and gently rocked him backward and forward until he stopped crying. The story goes that someone came in and found her with the baby and tried to snatch him out of her arms. Her screams echoed around the room as she tried desperately to keep hold of him, pleading with them to allow her to keep him. When a second person came to investigate the noise, she stood no chance and the baby was wrenched from her. She sank into a deep depression and died of a broken heart. They say that she walks the corridor and enters the room where her baby had been taken from her. Anyone who had ever been in that Victorian workhouse on a night when the windows rattle and the wind blows in straight off the sea, making a whistling noise, I think – even the most sceptical person – could be forgiven for believing that they could hear Jennie's screams. I wonder if anyone living in the new houses that have been built on the site ever thinks that they see or hear the sounds of Jennie crying for her lost baby.

Devonshire Road Children's Hospital was different altogether. It was the placement I liked the best. It was one ward on one level that was divided into three sections: the premature babies, older babies, and children up to eighteen years. The premature babies were so tiny and fragile. There were two of them that I still remember clearly. They were both boys. One tiny bundle was called Fred. There was nothing wrong with that, but it seemed such a hard name for such a small baby. It was also a very old fashioned name at the time. The other one had long black hair that went all the way down to his waist. Staff nurses wanted to cut the hair because it got in the way, but his parents were proud of it and wouldn't hear of it. When you looked into his cot, all you could see was a mass of black hair all over the cot; there was more hair than baby.

As in a lot of wards, the auxiliary nurse seemed to rule the roost. Priority had to be given to putting the clean linen away every day and keeping the ward tidy, but the most time-wasting task I was ever given was at this hospital. The clean terry towelling nappies all had to be refolded because the auxiliary did not like the way the laundry folded them. If it was that important, why didn't someone just ask the laundry to fold them lengthways in the first place? We were not allowed to nurse a crying baby because we were told it would 'make a rod for the mother's back' after the baby had been discharged, and she would not thank us for it. When the babies were fed, some nurses, instead of cradling them in their arm, kind of held them outwards, supporting the back of their head. It's as if they were too frightened of cuddling a baby.

A teacher came in two or three times a week to teach the older children so that they didn't get to far behind with their schoolwork. They didn't really do very much, but I suppose it kept them occupied, and like I already said, on the nice days we were allowed to take the children out for a walk. We had a motley assortment of beat up old prams. The deep-bodied ones held a couple of babies each, and we had some small trolleys that we could put the toddlers in. The older children just walked with us. We would put our capes on, and off we'd set. We all got a bit of fresh air. All these hospitals were in nice grounds, and we would walk around the gardens before go-ing into the cemetery next door. There was a lovely view if you looked over the gravestones and out to sea. The air was always bracing, and there were no complaints from the occupants. There was never any dog dirt; it would have been considered sacrilege to allow a dog to make a mess in a cemetery. The fresh air sharpened everyone's appetite and the children ate all their mince when we got back. Mince was served every day on account that that's what they ate the best they never seemed to tire of it. I loved the children's ward. It was decorated in bright colours and there was a large cupboard full of donated toys. There was also a supply of sweets, usually jellybeans, that were bought every week, and the children were given a few each day.

I also liked the P.N.H., the private nursing home back at the North Lonsdale Hospital, because they also had a maternity section. The young mums paid for an amenity bed, and that gave them a private room for themselves and their babies. I got to watch two births during my time on there; it was fantastic to actually watch a baby being born.

CHAPTER FOUR

When we reached our second year, and we went into 'block' (school), it was located in yet another Victorian building called Monks Croft, a house situated on the edge of town and originally built for the gentry. It was a large, imposing place, built in 1883 for James Thompson, who was a wine and spirit merchant. We all approved of this trade. The house stood in its own grounds, with its nearest neighbour being Priors Lea on one side. This was another mansion built for a civil engineer called Augustus Strongitharm. This house had also been taken over by the hospital authorities and was used for administration. It could be quite eerie at night. Ancient trees rustling in the wind and a long gravel drive meant that every little sound seemed amplified. The houses, in case you hadn't guessed by the names, were situated close to the ancient ruins of Furness Abbey, so this place was just about as isolated as you could get.

We always managed to walk into town but we often thumbed a lift back. One night Liz and I shared the back of a pick up truck with an enormous Alsatian dog after the driver stopped to offer us a lift. He assured us that the dog was quite friendly, and as sharing with a dog was better than the long walk back, we climbed into the back of the truck and sat as still as rabbits caught in the headlights. We hardly dared move a muscle just in case the dog thought we were its supper. It never took its eyes off us.

By this time, Ray and I had been meeting up quite regularly after bumping into each other in town again. We had been going out together for just over a year. He had a car, so I considered myself very lucky in that I nearly always had a lift back again. His car was a Morris 1000 called Betsey. It was hand painted blue and the wheel rims were red. If it rained, I had to brace my feet on the side of the car because the floor had a hole in it where the water came in and splashed my legs, kind of like the Flintstone's car. It had a crank handle that went in the front to start the engine. When it was being temperamental, and if it was raining heavily, he had to park it on a slope because we had to push it to get it started. I'll never forget those little wings that flipped up at the side as indicators. This was one up on winding the window down and sticking your arm out. When the wings got stuck, you had to clench your fist and bash the side of the car to encourage them to flip up. Ray had taken his driving test in Betsy, but alas it was raining that day, so Betsy was acting up. She conked out right in the middle of a junction. The examiner had to get out and push it until it got up enough speed to get started again. It wasn't all bad; Ray still passed his test.

The housekeeper at Monks Croft was not as strict with us as the home sister had been. She allowed us to stay out until eleven o'clock. Ray and I would usually sit in his car until the last student came in and then I would follow. This worked fine, until one night when the last one in was Dianne. As she disappeared through the door, I didn't realise she was rather the worse for drink. I knew she had seen me because she gave one of those soppy smiles that only someone who had drunk to much can give; her eyes were barely focused. I got out of the car and waved goodbye to Ray as he drove off down the drive. Then, as I made my way over to the door, all the drive lights suddenly went out and it was pitch black. I hurried over to the door, only to find it locked. Although Dianne had seen me, she was on automatic pilot. The last one in had to lock the door and put the drive lights out, which was exactly what she did.

It was cold and so scary. This house was the very last one, with only open fields and a few cows for company. There wasn't even a moon to help light the place up. I couldn"t possibly bang on the door and wake the housekeeper up. So, I started to throw some gravel up at the window of Diane's room, thinking logically that she would still be awake. She must have been dead to the world. I tried other windows but couldn't wake anyone. It had been way past eleven when Ray left, and as the time started ticking away, I got more and more desperate. If I didn't get to the loo soon, there would be an embarrassing accident. I had no choice but to hammer on the door. Finally, one of the windows flew open and a head popped out.

"Do you want to wake the housekeeper?" Dianne hissed.

"You've locked me out, you idiot", I shouted back angrily.

Just then, another window opened and Liz shouted down, "What's going on?"

Typical. It was like waiting for a bus, when there is not one in sight and then two come together.

"Will someone let me in before I freeze to death and wet my pants?" I asked.

I was so cross by this time. I had been out in the cold and the dark for nearly two hours. I didn't care who I woke up, but they did, and they dashed downstairs to let me in and keep me quiet. They made a big fuss of me and made me a hot drink to warm me up.

We didn't always have enough money to go into town. On these nights, we just talked or studied, caught up with the washing and such, but one night was different. We decided to hold an séance; heaven knows why but we did. We carefully made the letters of the alphabet and numbers one to ten and added two pieces of paper, one with the word 'no' written on it and the other with 'yes' written on it. We placed them in a circle around the edge of the table, and someone brought a glass from the kitchen and placed it upside down in the middle of the table. Just to add atmosphere, we turned the lights out and switched on a torch that was directed up to the ceiling.

We all placed one finger lightly on the glass in the centre of the table as I asked,

"Is there anybody there?" using my best and most mysterious voice.

I repeated this several times, when suddenly the glass started speeding around the table and then stopped dead. Everyone denied pushing it. Once again, putting on my best accent, I said,

"If anybody is there, give us a sign".

At that exact moment, the torch went out and we were plunged into darkness. Then we all heard a noise and felt a chill as cold air blew through the room.

'That's not funny", someone shouted. "Put the lights on".

When the curtains billowed out, we were really frightened. Someone managed to find the light switch and put the lights on. Then we all saw the settee move, and all six of us screamed in terror as we wondered what had we done. Who knows, we may have unleashed some terrible force. Then we heard it, faint at first, and then a quite definite titter. When a hand appeared on the back of the settee, we all froze, and then up popped the ginger head of Liz.

"Liz!" we all said in disgust. "What are you doing? You scarred us half to death".

She had been out for the night and was in a very merry mood. She had noticed the beam of light on in the living room and lifted the lower sash of the huge window that went all the way down to the floor. That's what had made the curtain billow out and had sent in the draught of cold air. The settee was in front of the window, and as she kind of rolled in, she pushed the settee out of the way. In a fit of giggles, she just lay there on the floor out of sight, not realising her muffled laughter sounded so eerie. We never did discover why the torch went out because when we tried it, it worked perfectly.

By this time, I had been working on the wards for about eighteen months and it seemed to me that some routines were set in tablets of stone, and no one ever queried why some tasks were carried out. One such task always puzzled me, so while in our second-year block, I did the unthinkable. I questioned the wisdom of the back round. The back round is no longer carried out, so let me explain what it was.

The back trolley had a stainless steel jug that held about six pints of water. Try lifting that when it's full. There was a stainless steel washing bowl and a stainless steel bucket, a stack of paper hand towels, talcum powder, a bottle of methylated spirit also known as surgical spirit, a tub of cream, and of course a bar of soap. The idea was to ask each patient,

"Do you want your back rubbing?"

If the answer was yes, they turned over on their side. It was more their bum that was rubbed, and I think that's why the men never said no. You lowered their trousers, carefully placed a paper hand towel underneath their bottom to protect the bed, and proceeded to pour a small amount of water into the bowl. Soaping up your hand, you gave their bottoms a jolly good rub. This was supposed to stimulate circulation, but as you could never get all the soap rinsed off, it seemed more like causing friction to me. You then dried the area and threw a liberal amount of talc over the skin, job done. This procedure was then carried out on the heels, except these were finished off with the 'meths'. It was suppose to harden the skin. The cream was for any sore areas, and as a lot of patients were confined to bed for long periods of time, the elderly in particular had lots of sore arrears. The dirty water was then thrown into the bucket on the bottom of the trolley.

This particular round always seemed so futile to me, and as was my nature, I voiced my opinion one day during class. You could have heard a pin drop as the class went quiet. The tutor looked at me, and then down at the floor, and then back at me as she struggled to find an answer. No one had ever asked this question before. I seemed to have flummoxed her. She carefully drew in a long, deep breath, and spoke in that kind of voice that is reserved for someone you are trying to placate, as though, maybe, that I was a few brain cells short of a brain.

"When the circulation is stimulated, it prevents bed sores", she said calmly and quietly.

"I think it creates friction and is a cause of bed sores", I persisted.

She just kind of glared at me and said, "I think we had better move on".

Well, that's all right, then. Question answered. I don't think so.

As we were now in our second year, we also had lectures from the consultants. I always looked forward to these, but at the same time kind of dreaded them. I blushed bright red if a stranger so much as spoke to me, let alone when I spoke to a consultant. They were right up there on the highest pedestal, right next to God – 'They', who must be obeyed without question.

So when Mr Silverton came to give us a lecture about melanomas, we all sat waiting for him to arrive with pens and notebooks in hand, trying to look intelligent. As he was about to begin, he seemed to be scrutinising everyone in the room. Then his eyes fell on me and stayed there. My face was so red I thought my head would explode. I wondered if I had left dinner around my mouth or something. Then he began, still not taking his eyes off me. I felt so uncomfortable. Then the reason for his attention became clear when he used me as an example of someone who may get a melanoma. He pointed out to the whole class my beauty spot, which he called a mole. 'That's charming", I thought. "How dare he call my beauty spot a mole". He advised that I should have it removed. Well, I didn't, and I'm still here forty years later to tell the tale. Then he slowly smiled as he said,

"I"m sorry. I shouldn't have said that, should I?" He was enjoying my embarrassment. For once, I never said a word.

We all loved being at 'Monks Croft', but the whole point of being there at this time was to sit the intermediate exams. It would be a big milestone in our training if we passed – our uniforms would then be changed to blue – but as well as passing the exam, we had to have a written report from the sister of our next placement. It was just my luck that I was sent to the female surgical ward on day duty for four weeks, followed by night duty for four weeks. Not that I minded the ward, but the sister had already had several arguments with my mother.

The serving of patients' meals was quite a ritual. Food was sent up from the kitchens in the dinner wagon, which the porters in their brown coats brought along to each ward. The dinner wagon was a large, heated, metal cabinet with an assortment of containers inside, each container full of different foods. There would be potatoes in one and vegetables in another. There was usually a choice from two dinners, but if they happened to run out of the one a patient wanted, it was Hobson's choice – take it or leave it.

When the sister was ready, the dinner wagon would be wheeled to the middle of the ward and all the nurses would queue up to take the dinners out to the patients as sister dished them. The special diets would be done first, which came ready dished from the kitchen. The specials would be: diabetics, who were allowed so many portions each day, and then there might be a low calorie, or a reducing diet as it was called, low protein, low/high fibre – there were all kinds of diets. Once these were given out, the full diets could have theirs: two scoops of mashed or boiled potato each – it was different each day – one spoonful of vegetables, and a serving of whatever the meat was. Nothing was frozen or pre-cooked; everything was fresh every day. Any patient who needed feeding was allocated a nurse for the job, who had to encourage the patient to try and eat everything on the plate, but who had to stand to feed the patients. The beds were all a fixed height, and once the patient was sitting up, you couldn't reach them any other way.

It was well known that some staff on some wards helped themselves to food that was meant for the patients. If it was leftover food, well okay, no harm done, but on this ward, on a regular basis, the domestic, or the pink overall as they were called, would be dispatched to the kitchens to ask for more food for non-existing new admissions. My mother, who was head cook and who had strong principles of what was right and what was wrong, had one day had enough, and she refused to give any more food without proof of new patients. When the hapless domestic reported back without any food, Sister Steel charged down to the kitchens like a bull after a matador. With nostrils flaring, she demanded to know just who did she, my mother, think she was – a mere domestic staff daring to refuse her, a sister in charge of a ward, the food she had asked for.

"You show me the extra patients', my mother said, "and I will give you the food".

It was like two bulls locking horns; neither would back down. Sister Steel eventually turned on her heels and stormed back up to her ward, shouting as she went,

"You haven't heard the last of this".

Well, she was dead right there, because mother hadn't finished with her either. She followed her up to the ward, drew herself up to her full height – all five foot two inches of it – and in front of the staff demanded to know where the extra patients were. Even old Steely hadn"t bargained for this. Oh! The nerve of this woman! In the end, she spluttered out,

"I had forgotten that two patients had been discharged, my mistake".

Smirking like the cat that got the cream, my mother returned to her domain in the kitchens. It was one of those peculiar class things of the day, when domestics and all ancillary staff where considered to be below the trained staff, and the two only talked when absolutely necessary. Domestics where there to be told what to do, and trained staff where there to do the telling.

Some years later, my mother told me the tale of a particularly snooty sister who walked into the kitchen one day and said, "Mrs Park, there's a rat on the roof". Quick as a flash, my mother replied, 'It's not my pet". I don"t know what she expected my mother to do with a rat that was running up and down the gutters, but at least now you can see where I get my big mouth from – or should I say, my sharp wit.

Anyway, I digress. You can see now why I was not happy with my placement. I was right to be concerned. I had finished my day duty and was reporting on for my very first taste of nights. It seemed a little strange that Sister Steel gave me my report in a sealed envelope when she was suppose to discuss it with me. She never looked at me once the whole time she was giving the handover report. As soon as she had gone, I dashed down to the sanctuary of the sluice to see what she had written. I couldn't believe it. Every grade was a 'D', and this included punctuality and neatness of uniform. I couldn"t help myself; I just burst into tears. How could she do this to me? It seemed so unfair. I had done nothing wrong, and no one had ever complained about my work. I must admit I should have watched my mouth a bit more and not questioned so many things, but I had never been late reporting on and I was meticulous about my uniform being just so. I never sat on my apron, and I was always careful to fold the corners up so as not to cause creases. This report meant that I had failed my intermediate exams and that I couldn't go into the blue uniform like everyone else from my group. I was heartbroken. I had worked so hard. Perhaps this was the point when I toughened up. I made the decision that this was wrong and I would say so.

I found it hard to work that night. Everyone knew something was wrong. That wasn't hard to figure out from my red eyes and 'sniffy' nose, and there was nowhere to hide either. On nights you sat at the ward desk that was positioned at the top of the ward so that you could see all the patients, with just one small light on so you could see to write the report. Unfortunately, that meant that everyone could also see me. I was assured that it was not the end of the world, but it felt like it. Everyone tried to be so nice to me, but the kinder they were, the more I cried. Eventually there were no more tears left, and in their place came a creeping dread that I had to give this report personally to the assistant matron, Sister Boyles, before going home in the morning.

Now Sister Boyles, the assistant matron, was half human and half Rottweiler. They tell me she had a softer side to her nature, but I was never privy to it. I was allowed to leave the ward a few minutes early in order to avoid Sister Steel. I did not want her to know how much she had upset me. I went along to the matron's office, with my heart in my mouth. Sister Boyles was like an oracle. She knew everything that went on in the hospital. She knew every patient"s name and diagnoses, and she certainly knew every member of staff. I went along to her office, my heart thumping, and tapped gingerly on the door. A voice called,

"Come in".

With my knees knocking together, I went in and handed over my report. She looked at it, and I waited for the rollicking that was sure to follow. As she looked up at me, her head tilted on one side.

"Why haven't you signed it, nurse?" she asked.

I summoned up all my courage and said, "Because I think it is biased, sister".

"Why do you think that, nurse?" she asked quietly.

"Well, for one thing, I've never been late, and I think I am always tidy", I blurted out.

Instead of the telling off I was expecting she just said,

"At the end of your night duty in four weeks time, get another report from the night sister".

That was it, no telling off. I think she knew about the argument that had gone on between my mother and Boyles, and she secretly backed my mother. She must have done; there was no other explanation.

I didn't sleep very well that day, but with all the support I got from my friends, I did feel a lot better. I was determined not to let Steel get to me. All the same, it was a relief that it wasn't Steel doing the hand over when I went to work that night. At the end of my four weeks of night duty, I got another report from the night sister. I had passed the intermediate exam. I was given the blue uniform and I never heard another word about Sister Steel's report.

The colour of hospital uniforms was very important. You could see in an instance what rank everyone was, from the pink overalls of the domestics to the brown coats of the porters. Doctors always wore white coats, except the consultants, and of course, there were the different colours of the nurses' uniforms: lilac, royal blue, and navy blue. It had been a very big deal for me not to get my new colour when everyone else did. I think the only uniform that has stayed traditional is the sisters uniform, which is still navy blue. Luckily, being on nights meant that I hadn"t met too many people who would notice that my uniform was not the same as the rest of my group, so most were none the wiser.

CHAPTER FIVE

Towards the end of my second year, just before Christmas, my placement was in the operating theatres. This was really daunting. I was looking forward to it, but at the same time scared stiff. Everything seemed to echo around the two theatres – the pink theatre and the green theatre. Everyone dressed in the same type of clothing. It wasn't so obvious who was trained staff and who was a student or a technician – they could have been anyone hiding behind those masks. My placement was for three months. For the first few weeks, all I seemed to do was clean out back, but gradually I was taught how to set the instrument trolleys ready for the operations, how to count everything that was used, and to check the instruments at the end of every procedure and mark each one on the board to make sure that nothing had gotten lost, or worst, left inside the patient.

I was allowed to watch the operations, at first from a distance, and then gradually nearer the table, being very careful not to get in the way. It never bothered me at all, whereas some students felt queasy when they saw their first operation, especially that first incision. In fact, I was more bothered by the smoke from the anaesthetic's pipe, which he never seemed to take out of his mouth. Even back then in the '60s, I could not understand why anyone was allowed to smoke over unconscious patients, or near any patient for that matter. My dad had always been very strict when it came to smoking. If my mother so much as smelt smoke on my clothes, I would get the third degree from my dad. He always said, "You're meant to eat so you have a mouth. You're meant to breathe, so you have a nose. If you were meant to smoke, you would have a chimney on your head". On the wards, the smokers often volunteered to tidy the sluice or the linen cupboard so that they could have a fag at the same time, but the most common place for a cigarette was the toilets with the window wide open.

Then came the day when I was allowed to assist at the operating table. I had been shown how to scrub my hands and lower arms, and how to put gloves on and 'gown up'. If you did anything in the wrong order, or fleetingly touched something that wasn't sterile, you had to go back to the beginning and start all over again. I did find it exciting and so rewarding doing a job that not everyone could do. I was glad I had stuck to nursing now and not left for better-paying jobs in the factories. I got quite a buzz out of doing this.

I really enjoyed my time in theatre. The only thing I didn't like was the fact that you were so closed in, with no windows, and no outside world for passing conversations. It seemed very much a closed shop, what we would call 'clicky'. If you were permanent staff you were in, but if you were only temporary, you were very much an outsider. As a temporary, you were not included in conversations until half way through your time there, when it seemed that suddenly they noticed you were there. There were times when it seemed as though you were treated as an alien.

Trouble seemed to follow me around, mostly because I spoke my mind. If only I could have held my tongue, life would have been a lot easier. While in theatre, one of the shifts you had to work for two weeks was the ghost shift. Basically, this meant that you worked a six-day week from four P.M. until midnight on five of the days, and on the sixth, which was a Wednesday, you started at six P.M. At midnight, you were not allowed to go home. You had to stay in the nurses' home to be on call for any emergencies. There was no pay for being on call. Really, there was no need for a student at all, but it meant a cheap way of having an extra pair of hands to be sent to any ward that needed help, and all the rest of the shift was spent cleaning walls in the theatre. It was really spooky to be there on your own. Everything echoed.

Even your own footsteps sounded like someone was following you, and of course you were a prime target for anyone who wanted to creep up on you and scare the living daylights out of you. Anyway, instead of doing just two weeks, I had to do four to cover for the other student who quite suddenly went off sick just as her turn came.

I thought what an unfair shift it was. I didn't get to see Ray at all because he worked until four thirty. I couldn't leave well alone, could I, so what did I do about it? Nothing too bad, at least I didn't think it was too bad. I wrote a letter to the *Nursing Times*, and I got lots of other students, over forty, in fact, to sign it. Well, you would have thought World War Three had broken out. The *Nursing Times* printed my letter, giving it a prominent position. My name, being the first, was printed, and then the editor noted that forty other signature accompanied this letter. The local paper saw the story and wrote an article about it, and in turn, the national newspapers repeated it. I was besieged with reporters phoning the hospital. Unfortunately, all the calls were either put through to my mother in the kitchens or the matron's office.

Oh, boy, was I in trouble! I even had reporters outside my house. First came the lecture from my dad, who told me in no uncertain terms that I should keep my nose clean while I was still a student. My dad went on and on and on, which was all rather puzzling, considering that my dad was a shop stew-ard who always spoke about work injustices and the rights of workers. Then came mother's input. She declared that I had brought shame on the family, and that she still had to work there, and that this would stay on my record forever. Everyone was talking about it. Finally, I was summoned to the matron's office, where both the matron and Sister Boyles sat with faces like thunder waiting to tear a strip off me.

"Do you consider this the best way to handle the situation?" I was asked.

If I hadn't written the letter nothing would have been done, but I didn't say that. I just kind of mum-bled,

"Maybe not, sister. I'm very sorry, sister".

"Three bags full, sister", I muttered under my breath.

It seems that this shift had been banned years before, but our hospital had kept it on and had been getting away with it until I wrote that letter. Well, some bigwigs descended on the hospital to investi-gate, and the shifts were stopped immediately. This made me popular with other students but not with the sisters. I did have to keep my head down for quite a while, and my dad added,

"For goodness" sake, keep your nose clean until your qualified".

This was the Christmas, in 1969, that Ray and I got engaged. We went to buy the ring during my lunch break. I had to get changed into civvies, or 'mufti' as we called it, before going into town. If I had been caught wearing my uniform outside of the hospital, I would have really been in trouble, and trouble was something I was trying to avoid, for a while at least. We had already been window shopping and had seen a ring that we both liked, so we went straight to 'Story's the Jeweller', where we were shown a tray full of rings, all sparkling under the lights. I chose the ring I had already seen in the window. We had decided to get engaged on Christmas Eve, but I couldn't wait that long for the official engagement. When we came out of the shop, I pleaded with him to let me have the ring now. We stepped into a shop doorway out of the rain, and he took the ring out of its little box, slipped the ring on my finger, and gave me a quick kiss, before he then drove me back to work. I rushed in to show everyone my engagement ring, holding out my hand so that the lights caught the tiny diamonds and made them sparkle. I couldn't keep it on at work, of course. The wearing of jewellery was strictly forbidden, so I pinned it carefully to the inside of my pocket, and for the rest of the day I was floating on air.

As this was Christmas, I would be able to wear it to the Matron's Ball. (It may have been the Mayor's Ball. I'm not sure, so I will call it the Matron's Ball.)

Every year, all hospital employees were invited to a ball. It was held in the town hall. All the ladies wore evening gowns and the men wore their best suits. There was a buffet and live music to dance to. It was a grand affair. It's a shame that such events are no longer held. It was the only occasion when all the staff got together and seemed to be equals, although there were quite a few 'catty' remarks to be heard, such as, "Look at her dressed to the nines. Who does she think she is?"

Matron's Ball was the highlight of Christmas. Local big wigs, including the mayor, also attended it. (Well, he would be there if it was at his invitation.) The group playing on stage would no doubt be called a boy band these days, but back then they were groups. On this particular occasion, the group's drummer worked in the administration office, and he was later to become the hospital secretary. They were really quite good, but there were a lot of older ones who would stick their fingers in their ears and complain, "It's so loud you can't hear yourself speak". Nothing's changed there then.

I've always loved Christmas, and Christmas at the hospital was no exception. Decorations were put up on Christmas Eve and taken down again on Boxing Day or the day after. Every ward had a real Christmas tree, and the week before had been spent making paper chains that the patients were only too eager to help with. Everyone went round the wards admiring the decorations. We were allowed to put tinsel around our caps, and on Christmas Day, a group of nurses, led by the matron, went round the wards in full uniform, including a cape and a couple of lamps for authenticity, to sing carols to the patients. During Christmas week, bands from around the town would come in and play carols. The Salvation Army Band, The Steelworks Band, and Vickers Band were just a few. I used to love listening to them. I don't suppose it would be politically correct these days for bands to play carols and nurses to sing, but to me it was magical and the patients loved it.

When the dinner wagons were taken to the wards, they were loaded with typical Christmas fare. There was a huge, freshly cooked turkey with all the trimmings. The dinner wagon would be wheeled into the middle of the ward as usual, only on Christmas Day, the ward sister would carve the turkey and plate each dinner individually, adding roast potatoes, fresh vegetables, and a chipolata sausage wrapped in bacon, all topped off with steaming hot gravy. Care was always taken when plating the dinners to arrange the food to look appealing, but on Christmas Day there was so much to fit on the plate that we had to be careful not to spill the gravy as we carried them over to the patients. After the dinner, for those who had room, there was a serving of Christmas pudding. Later on, at teatime, as a special treat, there would be freshly made mince pies, usually made by my mother.

The one other thing that marked Christmas as special was that a few days before would be the staff Christmas dinners. In groups of two or three sittings, the out-patient's hall was transformed into an informal dining room, set with tables that were decorated with crackers and tinsel. Paper streamers were hung up, and staff were served dinner by the ward sisters, home sisters, and matron. The men, mostly the doctors – there were not many female doctors then – porters, and ambulance drivers were all allowed a bottle of beer, and the ladies had a sherry. It was just so different from the strict routines that were followed every other day, it felt a bit like being Alice in Wonderland. After dinner, some of the junior doctors would sit on dressing trolleys or in wheelchairs and race up and down the corridors. It was all quite mad, and it was the only time when discipline was relaxed.

Our group was the first of the students to sit for the intermediate exams, which were taken at eighteen months instead of twelve months, as had been the practise previously. Then, once we had our new colour uniforms, we had to take on a lot more responsibilities, such as doing the doctors' round. This was always a daunting prospect, especially for me, as I still turned scarlet if a doctor so much as spoke to me. As second-year students, we were not quite up to doing a round with a consultant, but the more junior doctors still had to be accompanied. Mind you, it was often just as daunting for them, as the sisters' word was law. They wouldn't dare argue with her, and if she wanted something done, they did it almost without question, so often they were quite relieved if they went on a round with a student. Everything then was routine. It was the same type of operations, followed by the same treatments post-operatively. Patients were in for a lot longer than they are these days, and after anything major, they would be sent to a convalescent home. The main convalescent home for North Lonsdale Hospital was at Aldingham, which was right by the sea. A couple of weeks there was usually enough to build the patients up enough to go home.

On the medical wards, if I remember rightly, anyone who had had a heart attack, or coronary as they were always referred to, was put on six weeks bed rest. For the first two weeks, they were not even allowed to feed themselves. If they wanted a drink, a nurse had to hold a feeding cup for them. A nurse had to wash them, and when the bed was changed, the patient stayed in it, and he would be rolled from side to side while the sheet was put under him. Nurses had to lift him up onto the bed, and he even had to be lifted onto a commode once he was allowed to use one. Before that, they had to use bedpans. The nurse did so much repetitive lifting all day every day that the total weight lifted by the end of the shift could probably be measured in tons and hundred weights – and there was not a lifting gadget in sight. It beats me why there was so much surprise that a whole generation of nurses suffered so much with bad backs.

Patients got so used to being lifted that they would expect to be lifted, even when they were well on the road to recovery. I remember being told the tale of one rather large patient who wanted to get out of bed. He asked the nurses to lift him out, and it took four of them to struggle under his large frame. They managed to get him into a chair, made him comfy, and then carried on with their work. Once they had gone, he got up, walked around the bed to get his newspaper – you were not allowed to read a paper in bed on account of the print making the sheets dirty – and then sat back down again. He was asked why had he allowed the nurses to lift him when he was obviously capable of seeing to himself. He replied,

"But I'm a patient. I thought I had to be lifted".

I know this seems laughable now. Why on earth did the nurses lift him in the first place? But that's the way it was. Routines and customs were never changed.

After theatre came another few weeks in block, after which we entered our final year. During this time we worked a lot more night shifts, when we would be in charge of a ward. There were usually two other nurses to work with you and often a runner. This would be an auxiliary nurse who had to work between two wards. Night was so different from the day. The hustle and bustle had gone, all the back up had gone, and it was so quiet. Before settling the patients down for the night, the doctor, usually a houseman, did a ward round. The night sister also did a ward round, and she was there if there were any problems.

None the less, this was a lot of responsibility. There was such a lot to do, and I had to make sure it was all done. Medicines had to be given, drips needed replacing; whatever needed doing, I had to make sure it was completed.

The power of psychology is always surprising because back in the sixties, we were allowed to give out placebos, usually in the form of a vitamin C tablet. There were a surprising number of patients who could not sleep without their tablet. The tablet just happened to be vitamin C, but as long as the patient didn't know, they would sleep like a log, whereas without it they tossed and turned all night. Besides the responsibility of taking charge, there was one other thing you had to remember on nights, and that was not to switch the lights off in the kitchen because when you put them back on again the place would be crawling with steam flies and cockroaches.

My mother told the tale of one of the ladies who worked in the kitchen who one day was wearing open-toed sandals. When a cockroach crawled into her shoe under her toes, she stood there screaming for all she was worth. Sister Boyles just happen to be passing. She very calmly said,

"Get on with your work, and do stop that noise". Nothing ever fazed that woman.

One of the nights I have never forgotten was when a notice had been sent to all the wards saying that a plague of rats was being dealt with, but the poison being used was making them a little bolder than usual. We were to ignore any rats we saw because they would die in the end. On this particular night, I had gone on a message to a ward that had been added at a later date as a build on; it was well away from the other wards on the ground floor. On my way back, I nipped into a loo on a deserted corridor and was just about to sit down when I heard a faint splashing noise. Have you ever had that feeling when you don't really want to look but you know you have too? With my heart beating ninety to the dozen, I looked into the loo, only to see a rat swimming, doing the front crawl, or maybe it was breaststroke, I didn't stop to watch. I ran out of there, pulling 'me drawers' up as I went, and yes, I screamed like a banshee all the way to the switchboard.

At night you could always find a porter in the switchboard. With my clothes in disarray, he didn't know if I had been attacked or was having a fit. When I finally managed to tell him what had happened, he couldn't stop laughing. "Not very chivalrous", I thought, but he agreed to go back with me so he could see for himself. I had to go with him, not only to show him where it was, but also to stop him from flushing the rat down the loo. I couldn't bear the thought of killing an animal. I still can't. Yes, I know it was a rat, and I know I was stupid, but it was a living, breathing creature and *it* didn't know it was doing anything wrong. I pleaded with him not to hurt it, so he very gallantly stuck his hand down the loo in order to pick it up and put it out of the window. That ungrateful rat went and bit him. I had to write out an accident report and tell the night sister. I knew there was no way we could tell her the truth, so we had to make a story up of how he had dropped a pen behind a cabinet and as he squeezed his hand down the side the rat bit him. The poor porter had to have an injection of antibiotics and a course of tablets.

"That's the last time I'll do you a favour", he said, rubbing his backside where I had just given him the injection.

By now I had covered all the basic surgical and medical wards – paediatric, theatre, and geriatric nursing. Strange, isn't it, that only the name geriatric has been changed. Why not change the name 'paediatric'; it's quite similar in sound. Maybe we should say 'care of children' just to equal things up. Could it be simply the association with getting old? It won't be long before they change it again. Why use one word when four will do. I think it should be 'care of recycled teenagers'.

Anyway, to get back to the story, the ear, nose, and throat ward and the ophthalmic ward was right up in the attics. They were made up of lots of very small rooms, but I liked it up there because there were children. The wards were on two different levels, but at night they were run as one. It was on the E.N.T. ward that I learnt what a 'sarnie' was. Each afternoon, the patients were given afternoon tea, which consisted of bread and jam, and sometimes egg sandwiches and fresh cake from the kitchens. I had been a cadet when I was first asked to help make the 'sarnies'. I had never heard the expression before, and they all thought I was joking when I asked them how to do it. How was I to know it is just another name for a sandwich?

Each ward had its own coloured crockery that never left the ward. If pink plates were found on a ward that had blue crockery, they had to be returned. Sometimes while on nights, nurses would borrow a plate or cup, and then they would go on their brake, visiting a friend on another ward, and forget to bring the crockery back. Every so often, the most junior nurse would be dispatched to go round the wards, checking in the kitchen cupboards for missing dishware. Every ward had their own kitchen and a domestic who did the washing up. All crockery and cutlery was scalded after use using the deep sink that had an electric element at the bottom to boil the water.

Returning to the ward as a third-year student, I went on one night to find everyone in peels of laughter.

"What's going on?" I asked.

It took a while before anyone could answer, and even then it was between giggles as they all tried to control themselves. Finally someone said that they had asked a student to give a patient 'aminophilline' suppositories to help his breathing. When staff nurse went in a few moments later to check whether everything was okay, the patient was found with a suppository up either nostril that looked like a couple of torpedoes that were about to be launched. The poor man was really struggling to breathe.

"Are you sure this will help me breathe?" the poor patient asked, sucking in air through his mouth.

The staff nurse turned to the student and simply said,

"Other end, nurse".

It was all she could manage as she struggled to control her laughter. Well, you've got to admit that shoving something up someone's backside, and at the same time telling them it would help their breathing, does sound a bit weird.

Once we had finished our first third-year block – there were two blocks this year – we could then take charge of a ward, write reports, and take blood. This was usually on the 'regular' medical and surgical wards. I was sent to the gynaecological ward, which was back at the Roose site but in a separate building from the geriatric wards. This was a very big building for the number of patients there, again with lots of small rooms on two levels.

In block we had been given the task of writing a report, following a patient through from admission to discharge. I chose a girl who had come in for a late termination, or hysterotomy as they called it. I asked her permission and she said it was okay to write about her treatment. I knew this girl. Not only had she been one of my neighbours when I was growing up, but she had also worked as an auxiliary nurse. She was a bit younger than me. I went along to interview her for my report, and of course I asked her the reason for the termination. It seems the only reason was that she didn't want it. I tried not to show my feelings or be judgemental. After all, no one knows how they would react themselves if they found themselves in the same position, but I had to pursue this question because it was such a late abortion that she had to have a caesarean section. Her boyfriend left her the minute he knew she was pregnant, and she didn't know herself until the pregnancy was well on. I think by now she was about twenty-four weeks maybe a bit more.

Back in the sixties, it was still very much frowned upon to be an unmarried mother. There was never any mention that for every unmarried mother there had to be an unmarried father; they were considered to be Jack the lad sowing wild oats. If they denied being the father, there was nothing anyone could do about it.

When the time came to get Sally prepared for theatre, I asked her if she was absolutely sure of what she was doing. Times were changing, and she might be able to keep her baby and bring it up herself, or maybe send it for adoption, but she was adamant. She had thought about it, and this was the best solution, as she would have no support once the baby was born. She would be totally on her own. Once this was over, she could get on with her life. I took her to theatre and then got ready and prepared to watch. It only took a few minutes, but in that time her perfectly formed baby had been pulled out through the incision that had been made in her abdomen. It was plonked into a kidney dish, and I went over to have a look. My God! The baby was alive, and I shouted out,

"She's alive, she's alive".

The sister said,

"Leave it, nurse. It won't last very long".

I was so shocked that this tiny little girl had been put into a cold, metal kidney dish. Every instinct in my body cried out to give her a blanket, clean her up, and care for her.

"You can't leave her like this", I cried with tears streaming down my face.

She was taken away, and I was escorted from the theatre and told to go and get a cup of tea and pull myself together.

I could hardly look Sally in the face. The memory of her baby haunted me, and to make matters worse, I was told that babies' bodies were put in the incinerator, just something to be discarded the same as any other piece of rubbish – a human life, worth nothing. For Sally everything was fine; her problem had been dealt with. I'm not saying that she was wrong in getting rid of her baby. This was the swinging sixties, the era of love and peace. In fact, one of the favourite sayings of the day was,

'Make love, not war. 'Cause love is lovely, and war is ugly'.

But the older generation was still very much straight laced and could be very cruel. They could be hurtful and spiteful towards an unmarried mother, and there was not all the help available that there is today. I never saw Sally again once she had been discharged. I don't know how her life turned out without her baby. I wonder sometimes if she ever had children, and if she did, whether she thought about her first born.

While I'm back at the Roose hospital, I must tell you about William. He was a porter who had cerebral palsy. He couldn't walk a straight line, and we would watch him take the dinner wagons across the yard, zigzagging from side to side. We would bet each other if he would make it to the door without crashing. How he got through the doors at sixty miles an hour without hitting the sides is a mystery to this day. Okay, so it wasn't quite sixty miles an hour, but he did go fast and he never crashed, ever. He was an absolute marvel. He had a normal, intelligent brain trapped inside a body that wouldn't do as it was told.

William fitted right in at Roose. Nobody judged him. In the outside world, it was assumed that someone who walked like William and talked 'funny' must be 'nutty', and educationally sub normal. Everyone at Roose treated him like anyone else. To those who knew him, he was normal.

CHAPTER SIX

By now, Ray and I were looking at houses. We were to be married in October, in the week of my twenty-first birthday. We saw a house that we both liked, a mid-terraced, three-bedroom house with a bathroom. Well, not quite a bathroom, but a bath under the stairs and an outside loo. The bath had been hand painted with a white gloss paint that was peeling off. The house was rather expensive. At two thousand three hundred pounds, it was about three hundred pounds more than the average terrace. We got a mortgage for the two thousand, and we had to get an insurance to cover the other three hundred. The mortgage rates at this time were sky high. By the early seventies they had reached fifteen percent. There were so many people waiting to tell us what a mistake we were making. It would be like a millstone round our necks was a common saying we kept hearing, or that we would be in debt for the rest of our lives, but my dad always said renting is a mug's game. Always buy, and then one day you would own it; you never owned a rented house. His wise words have stood us in good stead ever since. So we started the long, drawn out business of buying our first home.

Meanwhile, back at the hospital, I had returned from Roose Hospital to work in casualty. I felt quite privileged because normally if you had worked in theatre, you didn't work in casualty. I absolutely loved it. There was all the excitement of theatre, but with the added bonus that you could talk to your patients. It was the mix I liked: male, female, young, old, medical, accidents – we covered them all. Casualty, like a lot of other departments, was made up of several rooms joined together, up a step here, down a step there. Part of casualty was the original theatre. It had an anaesthetic room, a sluice area, a preparation area, and two recovery rooms that were over on the other side of the corridor. It was a very small casualty, but then it only served the immediate population. There were lots of similarly small casualties up and down the country. Just about every town had its own. Things were so different back then. It's hard to start and explain, but I think that the biggest, most notable difference was the patients' attitude towards the staff. For the majority of people who attended, they were very genuine and very polite. There were some time wasters. Of course there were. They weren't perfect, but on the whole, people were grateful for whatever you did for them.

When I first walked in, I saw the couch that I had been laid on when I was a child. Well, a couch in the same position. I remembered my dad carrying me in after I had been flung off a round-a-bout at high speed. I was in agony with my injured leg. I couldn't walk on it. My mother had had to carry me home from the 'rec' – that's short for recreational playground where I was playing. Boy, did she struggle. She was only about five foot two or three. She had to keep stopping to hoist me up, as I was gradually sinking south. My dad was the first 'aider' at the docks where he worked, and he was in the St. John's ambulance. When he came in, he looked at my leg. It looked okay. There was no swelling, no deformity, and no bruising, but I was in agony, and I wouldn't let him touch it.

"We better take her to hospital", he said. "I don't think she's done anything, but it's best to be sure".

One of our neighbours had a car, and Dad borrowed it to take me to the hospital. Dad had laid me on the couch, and a big black man came towards me. I had never seen a black man in my life. I was ten years old. All I could see was a row of white teeth and the whites of his eyes. He didn't take the trouble to examine my leg. I can still hear him saying in a drawled out, funny accent,

"Oh, Sister! I was just going for my tea. Will you put a bandage on and bring her back in the morning for an x-ray?"

It was only five o'clock in the evening.

"Of course, doctor", she replied.

No one said a word to me. I lay on the couch with my teeth chattering together. It must have been the shock of the accident. My dad was told to bring me back tomorrow.

"She's alright", the doctor said. "She would be crying if there was any real damage".

"Thank you, doctor", my father said politely.

I don't know why he thanked him; he hadn't done anything. No one queried treatments. I spent the night in absolute agony, crying most of the time, and not knowing where to put myself. Every position was so uncomfortable. As the night dragged on, morning couldn't come soon enough. The next morning when I went back to the hospital, the same doctor saw me. He only spoke to my dad. As a child, I didn't exist, until he put his great big thumb on my leg and pressed hard where Dad had said it was sore. I certainly let out a yelp then. X-rays revealed a fractured tibia. No wonder it was so painful. I had to have a full-leg plaster cast on. The point being, my dad still said thank you and was grateful for the treatment I eventually received. He wouldn't have dreamt of complaining for the delay, even though it was two o'clock in the afternoon by the time I got the plaster cast on, and in all that time I wasn't given anything for the pain.

If anyone was abusive in casualty, the nurse in charge would simply call the police. No one stood for any aggression or violence. The police also came in handy for other things as well. Some patients, although violent, still had to have treatment – mostly drug overdoses, either accidental or intentional. If a stomach wash out was ordered, the patient could be particularly violent, during which time the porters helped to hold the person down, but if we still needed more help, or the porters were busy, the police were only too glad to help hold them down while the procedure was carried out. Actually, it was only a few years earlier that it was still against the law to try and commit suicide. The police would be notified in order to arrest them as soon as treatment was finished, or when they were well enough. Thank goodness this law was repealed in the early sixties so I never had to use it.

On the evening and night shift we still got our fair share of drunks – inebriates who could be aggressive or funny. One such man with a broad Liverpudlian accent came in after falling over and banging his head on the ground. The German doctor on duty asked him what was wrong with him.

"I've urt me 'ed, doc", said the patient in a broad, albeit slurred Liverpudlian accent.

"Vere is zee pain?" the doctor asked.

"In me 'ed", the patient replied with a mischievous twinkle in his eye.

This joke may be old hat now, but at that time it wasn't meant as a joke; it was just the way he spoke. I had never heard it before, and I found it funny. I tried to suppress a laugh that I could feel raising in my throat, but it only got worse. The doctor did not find it in the least bit funny, and as he sat down to scribble some notes on a card, my Liverpudlian friend looked up and asked,

"Was it your dad who bombed our chippy?"

That was it. I absolutely creased up laughing, and if matron herself had walked in, I would not have been able to stop. That was the first time I had heard that said, and I found it so funny; it was the best laugh I had had since the suppository incident on the E.N.T. ward. The doctor, on the other hand, did not find it to be the least bit funny. He walked out of casualty muttering something about the English and their strange sense of humour.

I liked casualty, and I didn't want to leave when my placement there came to an end. I didn't want to return to the routines of ward work. I knew already what kind of work I would like to do when I was qualified. Taking vases of flowers out of the wards at night or doing a shift of never ending rounds was not for me. I would like to work in casualty, where you never knew from one minute to the next what was coming in.

Now it was round about this time that I found out something that was to change my life. I discovered I was pregnant. This was catastrophic, not only because I had exactly nine months to go 'till I sat for my finals, and although I had not had any time off work, we were only allowed a total of six weeks off for sickness during our three years of training. It was still seven months 'till our wedding, but worst of all, how do I tell my parents? One thing was for sure: we had to bring our wedding forward from October. I had my pregnancy confirmed by my doctor, at six or seven weeks, and then we had to decide what to do. I mean, I could have just shot myself right then. Suddenly my final exams no longer seemed so important. They were right down on my list of priorities.

We resolved to tell my parents first, and then Ray's. We had arranged for Ray to come round one night when both of my parents would be in. We were not looking forward to it, but half an hour earlier, my dad had gone out and just my mam was in. Ray said that we should put off telling her until they were both together, but I didn't think my nerves could take any more, and anyway, he was only trying to dodge out of it; he was as scared as I was. We sat together on the settee and pretended to watch the telly, making small talk with mam. I kept squeezing his hand for him to start talking, but he didn't have enough courage yet. Eventually he said, "We've got something to tell you".

"Oh, yes?" my mam said.

"Er, um. Beryl is, er. Beryl's going, um …"

For goodness sake, I wished he would just get on with it. My stomach was so full of butterflies I hadn't been off the loo all day, and any minute now I would be going again. But there was no need to say any more. My mother screeched out,

"You're pregnant, aren't you?"

"Yes", I confirmed in a voice just above a whisper.

Well, that was it. She took a self-propelled rocket to the outer stratosphere, did a couple of circuits round the moon, and never landed on planet earth for several weeks. The names she called me – I hadn't heard of half of them – but the ones I had heard, well, they are unrepeatable. I mean the crime I had committed by getting pregnant was on par with murder, at the very least. She just sat there, not looking at me, and screaming every obscenity you could ever think of. Was it really that bad? Yes, it seems it was, and I knew it. This was the end of my world as I knew it, and I started crying.

"It's no good you sitting there crying", she screamed.

But floods of tears were not easy to stop. I was actually scared when Dad still hadn't come home and it was time for Ray to leave. I would be left to face him on my own. Thank God that by the time Dad came in, he was more than merry after having downed a few beers. At first, he started to make a joke of it, but Mother soon put a stop to that. I thought it best not to say a word. I quietly went to bed and left them to it. I thought I would face the music in the morning.

Our first priority, after telling his parents, who I must say took it much better than mine, was to rearrange our wedding. We brought it forward to June, rebooked everything, and then, just when we breathed a sigh of relief, we got a phone call informing us that the church had been double booked. We had to start all over again rearranging everything. In the end, it was rebooked for the fourth of July, the American Independence Day. We've heard every joke ever written about tying the knot on Independence Day.

The next few weeks were a mix of excitement and misery, as mam never missed an opportunity to get in as many sarcastic remarks as possible. She had quite an acid tongue, did my mother, in her younger days. Dad wasn't as bad as mam, but I had to sit through a lecture that went on for several days. Every time he thought of something else to say, he started all over again. Eventually things started to calm down, and I was eternally grateful that apart from a thickening waistline no one could tell I was pregnant until I was about seven months along, and by then I had been married for several months. I didn't have morning sickness either. I considered myself quite lucky,

B. Park-Dixon

as two of my friends, one of them Liz, were also
pregnant, but they put on weight early on, and their
pregnancies were obvious. As I was still only twenty,
I had to get the matron's permission to get married.
It was just a formality, but it had to be done. This
was another stressful duty I had to do on my own.
The matron probably knew, but said nothing about
a baby.

When Mam and Dad finally calmed down, they
started to help get the house ready and organise the
wedding. When the big day came, everything went
off perfectly. In case you're wondering, we did have
a big white wedding with a champagne reception. I
didn't see why I should miss out just because junior
was not exactly planned. We couldn't afford a hon-
eymoon because all our savings had gone into the
house, but we had two weeks off together and our
own home. What more could you want? We had
enough money to buy a three-piece suit and a fitted
carpet for the front room, a bed, and a cooker. Everything else that we had was given to us as wedding
presents – towels, crockery, cutlery, and bedding. We
had everything we needed. Our wardrobe consisted
of hanging coat hangers on the picture rails around
the bedroom until Ray had time to make some fitted
ones. We didn't have that many clothes anyway, so
we managed. I learnt early on how clever he was at
making things. I was very impressed as he set about
making stuff for the house. We were on the same

wavelength; any ideas I had he interpreted perfectly. My dad certainly admired his skills.

Back at North Lonsdale Hospital, I still hadn't told anyone except my close friends that I was to have a baby. There was no such thing as a maternity uniform, and my two pregnant friends had to wear huge white smocks. They looked hideous. At seven months, I asked for a larger uniform and that was all I needed.

I remember going over to the path lab, where I knew there was row after row of jars that held pickled specimens, by which I mean they were preserved in formaldehyde. There were brains, lungs – a healthy pink lung and a smoker's lung that was all black and covered in tar – as well as all the usual stuff. There was a row of foetuses at various stages of development, and right at the end there was a fully formed baby looking for all the world like it was asleep. I stood staring at them, trying to imagine what stage my baby was at, and how big it would be. In fact, foetuses look like babies from just a few weeks of development. They have all their fingers and toes. They may be tiny, but there is no mistaking a human life form.

One of my last placements was on the busy male surgical ward. There were four main wards at the hospital, each of which had had sun balconies added years ago. Originally, I think, they were meant to be used as a sitting area, but over the years, as specialities developed and the turnover of patients increased, the two on the surgical wards were turned into orthopaedic wards. The entire external walls were windows. As soon as the sun came out you were cooked, and even with every window opened, the heat could be quite overpowering in the summer. The few fans that existed were forever going walk-a-bouts. By this time, I was about seven or eight months pregnant and the ward was so full that extra beds had been placed down the middle. Usually, pregnant nurses were put on the smaller, quieter wards, and eventually I went to ask for a move, but there were no places, so I just had to stick it out. I only had two more weeks to go before I went on my twelve-week maternity leave – six weeks before the baby was due and six weeks after. I was totally exhausted. My back ached something rotten, and I knew I couldn't carry on if I stayed on this ward, so I went to see my G.P. He took one look at me and signed me off on the sick for the remaining two weeks with instruction to rest more.

Back at home, the nursery was just about ready. We had been given a cot, and everyone including myself was busy knitting baby clothes. I had bought twelve terry towelling nappies, along with half a dozen liners and a couple of pairs of rubbers. Apart from that, we were given just about everything a baby would need. People were only too glad to give all the stuff that their own babies no longer needed. My sister gave me her pram – a silver cross-coach pram – and my neighbour knit a complete baby layette, including a beautiful shawl. My mother and sister were both very accomplished on the old knitting needles, and they were clicking away every night until I had a fair mountain of cute little cardigans, hats, bootees, and blankets. One thing was for sure: this baby wouldn't get cold. We seemed to have just about everything. All we needed now was a baby.

CHAPTER SEVEN

The reason why I included my pregnancy in this tale was so I could include my experience of the maternity hospital. First the anti-natal clinic. I managed to keep most of these appointments, but I never went to any anti-natal classes because I didn't want anyone to know I was pregnant, and I hadn't been told about any, so I was none the wiser. At the clinic, there were three or four cubicles, and each one had a wooden bench across the back and a curtain to cover the front. Once changed into a hospital gown, you all sat together on a bench in a corridor. A nurse weighed us and checked our height in public – there was no privacy.

I think they were trying to make out that I was fat because they put me down as five foot three, which was three inches shorter than my height. All I did was point it out to them. I told them that there had been a mistake. They weren't too pleased when I asked them to change it. Strange that. It was a straight-forward mistake, but they didn't like me pointing it out to them. It seems they were annoyed because I shouldn't have been reading the notes. When they examined me, and for every examination after that, they told me how big the baby was. "Are you sure of your dates?" they kept asking me. Yes, I was dead sure, but now I was getting really worried that maybe I was having a baby elephant. Or, it could be twins, they said casually. Now that scared me, even though Ray is a twin. I knew they could only run in the female side of the family, but there was no scan to ease my fears. I think scans had been invented, but they were only used if the staff thought there was a problem.

I always remember that they asked me the date I got married. I should have told them to mind their own, but I told them the fourth of July and blushed bright red in the process. The exchange of looks between the staff may have just been my imagination – that knowing look on their faces. I hated being prodded about, and all those internal examinations. I had been told you loose all dignity when you become pregnant, and they weren't kidding. It was like a cattle market, but worse was to come.

We continued to decorate our house and try and save some money for a bedroom carpet. We didn't buy anything we couldn't afford. We saved for it first. We had decorated our bedroom orange, and all the bedding, blankets, bedspread, and eiderdown was also bright orange. Ye gods! When I think about it now, it's enough to give me nightmares, and there was more to come. When we finally had enough money to buy a carpet, guess what colour we chose? Why orange, of course. The only white in the room was the paintwork, and by now fitted wardrobes and a beautiful ottoman with a quilted top that Ray had made. I'll give him his due. He was clever, all right. He could make just about anything out of wood.

Ray was going to ask his dad to help him lay the carpet. By now I was about eight and a half months along, but I told him I was pregnant not ill, which is how I came to lift the bed out of the room and help spread the carpet out. I felt okay, although as the evening wore on I didn't feel too good. It was nothing I could put my finger on. I just thought I was tired, so I went to bed. I woke at two in the morning with an all-mighty pain. I thought, "This can't be it". My baby wasn't due for another two or three weeks. I waited for another pain, and, boy, it came all right – no half measures. I woke Ray up

"It's the baby", I said. "I think I'm in labour".

Now I've read stories where men go into a flat spin when their wives tell them they have gone into labour, and I've seen films where they go into panic mode. So how did my hubby react?

"Go to sleep. It's two in the morning" he said,

and he turned over. And that's exactly what he did: he went back to sleep.

I didn't know what to do. I didn't know what to expect. I couldn't even guess how bad these pains would get, so I got up and went downstairs and paced the floor for the next couple of hours. I had seen films when the mother to be screamed her head off. I wasn't up to that yet, but 'flippin eck', it didn't half hurt. In the end I went back upstairs and woke him up. I thought, "If I'm up, then he can get up as well". Talk about laid back; he still muttered,

"Are you sure? It's the middle of the night".

Now I have to admit that maybe I was getting a little short tempered; a bit tetchy, perhaps.

"Of course I'm bloody sure", I said, "and I know it"s the middle of the night on account of it being dark outside".

"Alright, there's no need to shout", came a sleepy reply.

Did I shout? I hadn't noticed, but at last I got a reaction. It was early on a Sunday morning at the end of November, and it was cold and dark. We now had the task of finding a phone box, with a phone that worked. I wasn't at all sure if I was ready to go to hospital, or if I should wait a while. One thing I was sure of was that you had to phone the hospital first, and you couldn't phone an ambulance unless it was an emergency. Being in labour was not an emergency. I prayed that the car would start. It didn't, but luckily it was parked on a short slope. Ray turned to me and said,

"Hey, B. Can you give us a puuu … Never mind", he added hastily.

He was about to say could I give that perishing car a push, but one look at me reminded him that I was about to have a baby, and I was in no mood or condition to be pushing a car, so he quickly changed his mind. Boy, he sure made the right decision, 'cause I think I might have just killed him if he'd had asked me to push that car. We found a telephone box and phoned Risedale Maternity Hospital. They insisted on speaking to me, but I was in the middle of another contraction and I was scrunched up on the floor. Ray held the phone to my ear.

"They want to speak to you", he said in a very matter-of-fact way.

"Yes?" I snapped.

"How far apart are your pains?" they asked.

I felt like saying they weren't far apart at all, that they were all in my belly, but I didn't.

"Ten minutes", I gasped through gritted teeth.

"How strong are the contractions?" was the next daft question.

How the heck did I know what was considered strong? I mean, I thought I was dying. "Is that strong enough?" I asked sarcastically.

"Well, if it's your first, you'd better come in, but I doubt that you're in labour. It's too early, and the first baby is nearly always late".

Well, someone should tell that to this baby because it sure felt like it was about to come now. I wasn't reassured. It sounded like they didn't want me, and if it wasn't labour, what the heck was it?

We arrived at the hospital and rang the bell at the side of the huge wooden door. It seemed like an eternity before anyone answered it. Finally, the door swung open.

"You must be Mrs Dixon", said a voice. "Say goodbye to your husband", she said as she took my case off him.

His feet didn't even get over the threshold. Before she slammed the door shut she told him,

"You can phone in later. Give it a few hours. I don't expect this baby to come any time soon". And with that, he was gone. The door shut with a bang. I knew that husbands were not allowed in with their wives, but I thought he would have been allowed in for a few minutes. It's not as though I wanted him in the labour room, although I had heard that in the bigger city hospitals some husbands were actually staying with their wives and watching the birth. Now, personally, I think that's taking things a bit too far. I'm absolutely positive he would have ended up passing out, sprawled on the floor, being more of a hindrance than a help. Or maybe I would have thumped him just because of the pain I was going through.

I followed the nurse up the corridor into a room with an examination couch and a table, where she put my case, and in a small adjoining area, there was a bath and a toilet. I suppose that would be called an 'en suit', but I don't think the word had been invented yet. She told me to get on the couch and she prodded my bulging stomach.

"Well", she said. "You'll still be here this time tomorrow".

"Oh, great", I thought. "Does that mean these pains are going to get worse?"

She ran a shallow bath and poured a copious amount of Savlon into it, with the instruction that I was to have a bath and take my time, as they were busy and I was a long way off having my baby. She disappeared out the door and I was left on my own. It was so quiet. There wasn't a sound. I must have been a long way away from anyone else. I found all this very frightening. I didn't think these pains could get any worse. The last thing I felt like was a bath. I gingerly got into a two-inch deep puddle of anti-septic, tepid water. I quickly got out again when the suppositories that had been shoved up my rear end started to work. I would have been given an enema but for the fact that I had had diarrhoea for the last ten hours, so there wasn't much left inside me.

When she finally came back, I was taken into a labour room that I was to share with another woman. Shortly afterwards an auxiliary nurse came in with my breakfast. Is there any woman in the whole wide world who could eat food while in labour? I was told I had to eat because I would still be here this time tomorrow, and I would need my strength, whereas the woman next to me was told to eat a little if she could manage it, as it wouldn't be long for her now. What a cheery lot they all were.

A midwife came in a couple of times during the morning, and my roommate was given a tablet for the pain. I asked if I could have something. "It's going to get a lot worse yet", she said, but she gave me two tiny blue tablets. I looked at them and thought, "These look an awful lot like phenergan. What good were they going to be?" They were an anti-histamine, so weren't they meant to treat hay fever? I was in no position to argue. I took them, grateful for any little thing that might help. By eleven o'clock, the midwife had still not even looked at me. She was only interested in my roommate, who spoke with a plum in her mouth. She was a lot older than me. She must have been in her thirties at least. Poor lamb, I don't see why her pain was any worse than mine. It crossed my mind that I might be delivering this baby myself for all the help I was getting. I did think I should give an almighty scream and then sit back to see if I got any attention. I didn't, coward that I am, but when once again my roommate was being checked over, I could actually feel my baby coming. I asked the midwife would she mind looking at me. Okay, so I was pleading, but by now I was getting desperate. I really couldn't take any more pain.

"There's not much point. We really are very busy", she said.

"Please", I pleaded. "I can feel it coming".

I can't remember what she actually said, but it was something like,

"You silly girl, you're not ready yet".

But she did stop and take a look at me. The time was five past eleven. Instantly, she changed her attitude towards me. She rang a bell and instructed the auxiliary to walk me to the delivery room. The rotten sods, walk! In my condition? I kind of shuffled along the corridor, holding onto my belly. It felt so heavy. One thing was for sure, they certainly didn't believe in molly coddling you. I kept thinking the baby was about to drop onto the floor. Luckily he didn't, but when I finally got to the twin delivery room, my heart sank. There were two beds facing each other. I mean, would it have done any harm to give us just a little bit of privacy? I must admit I was a bit past caring. I just wanted to get it over with.

A thin curtain divided the beds. Lucky for me, my roommate was not about to have a baby any time soon, so at least I had the delivery room to myself. I got on the couch and lay on my side, clinging onto the rails of the bed every time another wave of pain came. Then I felt a sharp needle in my leg, and at the same time a doctor 'released' my waters. Great, no one thought to tell me anything. The first I knew what was going on was when I felt the extra pains when the needle went in and the scissors cut me. The needle was the long overdue Pethidine for the pain. I got the feeling that the whole process was like being on a conveyer belt – examination room, followed by the labour room, next the delivery room, and after that, hopefully, a nice, comfy bed in a ward. It was very strange. I couldn't shout or scream like they do in the films, instead, I made a 'mmmm' sound from the back of my throat that sounded a bit like a cow mooing. I know I ended up with a sore throat. Someone kept trying to give me gas and air, but I couldn't let go of the bed rails I was clinging onto, so I couldn't hold it.

"You'll get a sore throat making that noise", said one wise old owl.

How come all the midwives seemed to be spinsters who had never had any children? "Stop pushing", someone kept saying. There seemed to be so many people around me I couldn't tell which one was speaking, but I wasn't pushing. It was coming all by itself. Whether they liked it or not, this little beggar was fighting his way out. He didn't intend to stay in there any longer. Anyway, thank goodness it didn't go on too long. The elephant I thought I was having was in fact a five-pound, twelve-ounce baby boy who was born at eleven thirty-five A.M.

I was ecstatic. This was the first boy born in either family for ages. Ray had three sisters, one of whom had a girl, and I had one sister who also had a girl. I couldn't get the grin off my face; I was beaming from ear to ear. A boy! I couldn't get over it. I was crying and laughing at the same time.

"'Ere, look at this 'un", someone said. "What you crying for?"

I just ignored her; no one could burst my bubble. I was allowed to hold him for a few seconds, and then he was whisked away.

Now normally, I understand, you were left to lie on these trolleys for several hours, but it seems dinner was being served and I had to eat some. They were so hung up on food. So, I was taken to a bed and given a salad. Unfortunately, I had been awake all night and the Pethidine was just kicking in. As soon as I got in bed I fell asleep. A few minutes later, I was shaken awake.

"Mrs Dixon", said a voice. "You must eat your dinner to keep your strength up".

Here we go again: me and my strength. They must think I need building up or something. I looked up into the stern face of an auxiliary. The auxiliaries seemed to rule the roost in all the hospitals.

"I want to sleep", I murmured.

"You must at least eat the protein", she said. "Eat the egg and a bit of meat". She stood back with her arms folded across her ample chest and glared at me until I had eaten what she said, but that wasn't the end of it. As I started to fall asleep again, she once more shook me awake.

"You have to drink a glass of milk".

For goodness sake, all I wanted to do was sleep. I knew that if you fed your baby yourself you got a free pint of milk a day. Now I like milk, and normally drinking it would have been no problem, but I was so tired that all I wanted to do was sleep. I managed to drink all the milk, and at last I was allowed to go to sleep, but not for long.

CHAPTER EIGHT

On a Sunday, visiting was in the afternoon. Visiting hours were very strictly adhered to, and just before the visitors were allowed in, the ward became a hive of activity. The beds had to be straightened and the ward tidied before anyone was allowed in. I could see the visitors waiting outside the doors, and right at the very front I could see a huge bunch of flowers that seemed to be topped off by a head of thick curly hair. The Chrysanthemums obscured the face, but I'd recognise that head of hair anywhere. Who else could it be but Ray, proudly holding the flowers high. He was first through the doors. He told me that all the other dads had been asking where he got the flowers from on a Sunday, as no shops were open. He had been around the allotments, asking his dad's mates if they had any flowers because his wife had just had a baby. They were as pleased as punch, and after giving hearty congratulations, obligingly picked their best blooms. His grin was as wide as mine.

My baby hadn't been brought back to me, but Ray had been allowed to look at him through the nursery window. It was Ray who told me how much the baby weighed. No one had told me. He had been taken away and put in the nursery because of his low birth weight.

Not many people had a telephone in their house, so Ray, poor thing, in order to keep a check on my progress, had to go to the pub to use the phone. Well, that's what he told me. He didn't want to use a public phone because he didn't know how many times he would have to ring, and he didn't want to use his parents phone because the pub was more appealing, hence the smell of beer when he came to visit.

After visiting, I couldn't wait to get some sleep. The only thing was, after the birth I was so thirsty I had drank gallons of water. I was probably parched from all that mooing I did. Okay, so I exaggerate a bit. Maybe not gallons, but I did drink several cupfuls, and now all that water had to come out at some point. My point was in the middle of the night, but I wasn't allowed out of bed so I rang the bell. It seemed an age before anyone came. I thought, "There's going to be a flood if they don't hurry up". Eventually a voice said,

"What do you want?"

"I need the loo", I said apologetically.

She grudgingly said she would get me a bedpan, and she returned just in time with the curt instructions,

"Lift up".

It was such a relief. When I'd finished, I rang the bell again. It was the same auxiliary.

"What is it now?" she snapped.

"I've finished", I said meekly.

"Can't you get yourself off?" she asked as she yanked the pan out from under me and put it on the chair by the bed.

"Sorry", was all I could mutter.

Sleep seemed wonderful, but it couldn't have been more than half an hour before I woke up needing that dreaded pan again. I was too frightened to ring the bell straight away, and I waited as long as I could, but needs must be met, and when I could wait no more, I plucked up the courage to ring. It was just my luck. Godzilla came back.

"What do you want now?"

Flipping 'eck. I don't know which charm school she went to, but I bet she failed the course.

"I'm sorry, but I need the loo again", I whispered, frightened of waking everyone up. "I've held it as long as I could, but I can't wait any longer".

Fancy having to apologise because you need to wee. She pointed to the half-full pan on the chair and said,

"You've got a pan already".

"But it's been used", I said in astonishment, my whispers getting louder.

"Well, you can use it again, and when you've finished, put it back on the chair. Lift up".

Alas, when I'd finished it was so full there was no way I could take it out myself. Now I was in a right pickle. What could I do? I sat there in the dark, perched on the 'throne', trying to weigh up my options, but it was no good. I would just have to ring the bell again. Much to my relief, another nurse came.

"Do you need a hand?" she asked pleasantly.

"Oh, thanks!" I said, taken by surprise at hearing an agreeable voice.

"It's a bit full", I volunteered.

"My, my! You must have been bursting", she said as even she struggled to avoid an overflow.

"You're not kidding", I replied, "but there are two lots in there".

It was nearly morning, and thank goodness I didn't need any more bedpans, but you could have knocked me down with a feather when, first thing, Godzilla returned, stood at the top of the ward, and adopted her now familiar pose of arms across chest. Starting with me, she shouted down the ward,

"Mrs Dixon, go to the toilet".

I didn't need to go. I had done enough in the night, so I started to say,

"It's okay, I don't need to go, thank you", but Godzilla was adamant.

"Mrs Dixon, would you please go to the toilet?" she said in a voice that was not to be argued with. I haven't been instructed to go to the toilet since I was about five years old, but I thought it best not to make a fuss, and I got out of bed and put my slippers and dressing gown on and started to walk towards the bathroom.

"Right. That's okay, Mrs Dixon. You can go back to bed now. I just wanted to see you walk".

Well, why the heck didn't she say that?

The wards here were not like the North Lonsdale wards. They were called bays, and each bay had six or eight beds in it. When they brought the babies in after breakfast, they walked to the top of the bay and just shoved the cribs in the direction of the mother's bed, shouting the name as they did. Each crib free-wheeled until it came to a standstill somewhere close to the bed. I waited for mine with that big soppy grin on my face, full of expectation of what it would feel like to give little junior a cuddle and hold him for as long as I wanted. After all, I had only seen him for a few seconds the day before. However, you didn't need to be Einstein to count only five cribs and six mothers. Where was mine? I started to feel panicky, as I was the new mum without a baby.

"Where's mine?"

"Your what?"

"My what? My baby of course".

"Oh, it's in the nursery".

"Why? I want to see him. I only saw him for a few seconds yesterday".

"Don't panic", said the midwife. "I'll see what I can do".

She returned a few moments later with this tiny, blond-haired, sun-kissed baby.

My reaction was instant.

"This one's not mine. Mine had dark hair".

She quickly took him away again, but within a minute returned, saying,

"There's no more left. You'll have to have this one. The other Mrs Dixon had a girl". She smiled. "You probably saw him with wet hair that made it look dark. Once it's dried and cleaned up, it's blond".

Phew, that's a relief, but it didn't explain the suntan. That, too, was easy to explain. Apparently, he had been born a bit jaundiced, which made him look yellow. I instinctually went to pick him up.

"Now don't you be nursing him all day. You'll make a rod for your own back and regret it when you get him home".

Every nurse seemed to say these pearls of wisdom, but as I didn't agree with them, I picked him up anyway. I was a mother! I could hardly believe it. This tiny little bundle was my son.

I didn't sleep very well in here, on account of the thick rubbers on the beds that made me sweat. After two nights of tossing and turning, I decided that enough was enough. The rubbers would not be removed until four or five days after birth. I carefully took the rubber off and, folding it neatly, hid it under my pillow, replacing the draw sheet so that it wouldn't be noticed. When the day came that it would be removed officially, I put it back on again. No one was any the wiser, but I got a decent night's sleep.

I had ten days in here, which was the standard length of time after having a baby, but I couldn't wait to get home. Ray came every visiting time and sat there resting his chin on the edge of the crib, staring at the tiny infant, who didn't seem to do anything other than sleep. The infant, that is – not Ray. I found out the reason why he was so sleepy. He had been put on medication because of the jaundice. No one had thought to tell me, and of course that was the reason why he seemed to have a lovely suntan – it was the jaundice. He had been put under a sun lamp for twenty-four hours when he was first born, which is why I didn't get to see him until the next day.

When my ten days in Risedale Maternity Hospital were finally up, Ray brought in the bag I had already packed with a new little baby grow, a hand-knitted cardigan, a vest, a terry towelling nappy, and those invaluable rubbers, not forgetting a warm shawl to wrap around baby to keep out the autumn chill. Everything for the baby was provided while we were in the maternity home; you were not allowed to use anything from outside. I was given a free Milton steriliser and baby bottles when I left. Not everyone got one of these, but the company sent so many every week and they were given randomly to the mothers. I happened to be one of them.

All the new mums were also shown how to top and tail the baby. They always use to show the mums how to bath baby, but there was some reason or other why they couldn't do that, so the midwife told us how to hold the baby securely while bathing it by using a doll to demonstrate. Then we were taught how to swaddle them in a shawl or blanket. The idea was to make the baby feel secure as well as warm, so that they would be more contented. Finally, we were shown how to wind the baby after each feed. That was it; all the basics covered.

When the time came for us to leave, it had never occurred to me that my normal clothes would not fit me. When I took out the trouser suit that I had packed for myself to go home in, I really could not understand why I couldn't fasten the trousers up. It was so embarrassing. I had to ask for some nappy pins that I linked together to form a chain to loop through the button hole and across to the other side to hold my trousers up. At least the loose top covered the pins. A midwife carried the baby to the waiting car parked by the door. After I got in she handed him to me. I said a silent prayer, hoping that the car would start, and it did. We were on our way home at last. Now, the hard work would really begin.

I had eight weeks of maternity leave left. My final exams didn't seem so important now, but I had to go back to work for at least three months, otherwise I wouldn't get the last month's maternity money, which was kept back just to make sure I returned to work.

CHAPTER NINE

I spent every spare minute I had swotting up on all the work I had done so far, but I didn't have much time with a new baby in the house. It was surprising how much washing this tiny little thing could make, and with no washing machine or spin dryer, it wasn't easy to keep on top of it. The bath being right next to the kitchen came in handy for soaking the washing. Then, after a few hours, I would take my shoes off and in bare feet I trampled the washing, walking up and down the bath 'till the water looked suitably dirty. It was quite therapeutic, really. It was all rinsed in much the same fashion; the hard bit was the ringing out. On the large items like towels or sheets, Ray would hold one end and I would hold the other, and we would twist the washing in opposite directions until we squeezed out as much water as possible. Then I would string a line across the back street and hang it out. Just about everyone did their washing on a Monday because no coal lorries came down on that day. If any other lorry driver dared to risk life and limb going down a back street full of washing, the call went out from house to house: "A lorry's coming", and everyone would run out and grab their washing lines and scowl at the driver as he drove past. I had to keep up with the nappies, though, as there was only twelve. They were put to soak in a bucket and then washed by hand every day.

Anyway, housework aside, in the evenings, once the baby had gone to sleep, out came my books, and with Ray struggling to pronounce half the medical words, he sat testing me, asking questions about nursing. The days went quickly, and before I knew it, it was time to return to work. This was the hardest time of my life, to leave a new baby who was only eight weeks old while I returned to work. It was touch and go whether I would go back or not, but Ray convinced me that I would regret it if I didn't give it a try. After all, it was only for three months. It was with a heavy heart that I returned, but it wasn't as bad as I had thought because I returned on the same day as Liz. She had had a baby the day before me, so we could talk babies and compare notes for the extra study we had been given and play catch up together.

Now, we were supposed to be given a refresher course, but when we inquired about it, we were just given a blank stare and told that there was no such thing. We would just have to organise ourselves, and revise what we thought was the most appropriate.

It was very hard work getting a baby ready at six in the morning before work to take to my mother-in-law, who was looking after him, get myself ready, and actually get to work, do a full shift, return home, collect junior, keep up with the washing, look after a baby, and try to study. There were so many times when I thought it just wasn't worth the hassle, but Liz and I carried on together. By now, we had been put in the class of students behind us, and when the time came, we sat our finals together at Lancaster. We had to do a practical exam and a written exam. We had done mocks and practised things like setting a dressing, trolley aseptic techniques, and lots of other everyday nursing procedures.

On the morning of our practical we arrived early at the railway station to catch the train to Lancaster. We were so nervous. On the train, my stomach felt like it was full of butterflies. We spent the whole journey asking each other questions. We had spent three years preparing for this, and we were about to find out if it had all been a waste of time or not.

When we got to the hospital, we were suppose to report to the practical room in the school of nursing, but we couldn't find it, and there didn't seem to be anyone else around to ask. In fact, the place seemed deserted, and we started to doubt that we had the right day or even the right place. Finally someone appeared, and we were given instructions to go straight to the classroom, as we were nearly late. Of course it just had to be on the other side of the building on a different level, but first we had to get changed into our uniforms. We finally arrived, all neatly dressed, with shiny shoes and tied-back hair, with flushed cheeks and heavy breathing, because we had had to run. I thought that any minute now I was going to be sick, I was so nervous.

We were given a few minutes to familiarise ourselves with the layout of the room and the equipment. Everything seemed so different. I had thought that all hospitals used the same packs, such as a dressing pack. Ours had everything in them that was needed to do a dressing: two little galley pots – one for Savlon and one for Hibitane – and swabs, all set on a foil tray, and the whole lot parcelled up in a large paper that was used as a sterile field. Here everything was sterilised individually and you had to make up your own packs.

There were two examiners, and of course we were not allowed to talk to each other. A voice called out that the exam was about to start, and we each went to the opposite ends of the classroom. Trying my best to look confident, I stood in front of the examiner and listened intently to the task he was setting me. It was quite strange really. It sounded like his voice was a long way off, coming through a mist. Or was that my brain just fogged up?

He told me that I was to prepare a trolley for bilateral traction for a dislocated inter vertebral disc. My God. I'll never forget it. I didn't have a clue what he was talking about, and I could feel a rising tide of panic overwhelming me. I tried to calm down. "Now think", I told myself. He had mentioned traction. I could do that. And he had mentioned vertebra, so it had to be orthopaedic. I grabbed a dressing trolley and headed towards the weights and pulleys and frantically started to almost throw the stuff on the trolley. Oh, how I wished I had slowed down and been a bit more careful. Too late, as I pulled at the set of weights, and they all fell off the metal rod that held them. Our weights had a hole in the middle and they just slid down over the rod. These, alas, had a gap through the side and they were, well, just kind of slipped in place and precariously balanced. The noise was unbelievable as they crashed to the ground and rolled in every direction. Before actually coming to a standstill, they seemed to spin for an eternity before finally falling flat. I was so embarrassed as I ran around the room trying to get to them before they went into a spin, my face bright red. I caught a glimpse of Liz's sympathetic look, and then the volunteer patient, who was trying to suppress a laugh with his hand over his mouth and his shoulders going up and down, and then the examiner, expressionless apart from raised eyebrows, who just stood there looking at me. I suppose I was lucky, really, if one of the heavier weights had landed on my foot it could have broken a bone. I mean, I could have ended up crying as well as embarrassed. As it happened, the examiner said,

"You can leave that, nurse. It's obvious you know what you're doing".

Do I? Well, of course I did. I was only kidding when I said I didn't have a clue. Phew! This was the worst possible start I could have imagined. The rest of the exam didn't seem to go that well either. When it came to the oral questions, he asked what kind of nursing would I like to do. I thought he was trying to put me at ease. Foolish me, it was a trap. I replied,

"Children. I love working with children".

"What about geriatrics?" he asked without commenting on my reply.

"No. I really like children", I insisted.

He was having none of it.

"Both groups of people need care; they both need keeping clean and fed", he persisted.

I felt like saying there's a bit of a difference in changing a baby's nappy and changing an incontinence pad, or that I could hardly sit an eighty year old on my knee and bounce him or her up and down. I didn't say any of that, of course. I only thought it. I agreed that both groups of patients, in fact any patient, needed the same basic care, but that I preferred children. He spent so much time on this one question, which actually did nothing to test my knowledge of nursing, that I only had a couple of questions before the time was up; he would not give up on it, which is why I felt so down on my way home. There was no way I could have passed. It must have been dropping those weights right at the start that maybe put him in a bad mood. Whatever it had been, I knew that I had failed.

It was with a heavy heart that I told Ray I didn't think I had done very well in the exams.

"It doesn't matter", he said. "At least you've given it your best shot".

My tutor came looking for me the next day to ask me how I had got on. I wasn't worried about the written exam, but the practical had been particularly nerve racking when the examiner kept going on about geriatric and paediatric nursing being the same. Even the tutor agreed that it had been unfair to pursue a question I had already answered. Anyway, there's nothing I could do about it now. I still had the rest of my twelve weeks to work, at the end of which I had to officially give in my notice, but I was still asked what kind of work I would like, and what hours would suit me. Everyone, and I mean everyone, was offered a job. No one ever took their finals and was then told that there was no work for them. It was all a bit deflating, really. This was what I had worked towards since the day I left school, but at the end of it there was nothing. There was no way I could work. Well, not yet anyway.

Which just about brought me up to the present day. I was jolted out of my daydream by my husband's loud question.

"Beryl, will you open that letter or I will open it for you?"

Full name, he must be getting impatient.

"Okay, okay", I said as I carefully opened the letter. I read the first few words:

"It is with pleasure".

"Yes", I shouted.

There was no need to read any more; I had passed. Well, did you ever doubt that I would pass first time? Now I had the best of both worlds: a beautiful baby and my qualifications. I could now legally call myself an S.R.N. – a State Registered Nurse, a staff nurse. All the hard work had been worth it. Then I was brought down to earth with a bump as I realised that I would be leaving work to look after my baby.

The next day I went to matron's office to tell her my good news. It was Sister Boyles whom I spoke to. She immediately offered me a job in the isolation unit at Devonshire Road Hospital. Everyone was always offered a job; no one was made redundant. I was offered part-time work with hours to suit me. I was so excited at passing that I didn't want to leave, and I talked it over with my husband when I got home, but it just wasn't practical to leave such a young baby. Plus, how was I to get there? It was at the Devonshire

Road hospital, and I didn't drive, so I reluctantly re-fused the job and handed in my notice.

Two and a half years passed by, during which time I had a second baby, a little girl born on the fourth of July – yes, our anniversary. We had moved to a bigger house and I had passed my driving test. It was after we moved that I started to get restless all day and my thoughts turned towards nursing and my longing to return to work. I had to figure out a way that would allow me to return to work that would still leave my days free to look after the children.

I hardly knew anyone in the new area we had moved to, outside of family, that is. We had moved close to where I had been brought up, so my sister was close by, as were my parents, but there was no one to baby sit, and all day long all I heard was baby talk. I was going stir crazy for adult conversation and I needed something to occupy my brain. I hadn't done all that training just to stay at home and not practise. So, with that in mind and without saying a word to Ray, I wrote to the hospital asking if there were any jobs on the granny shift, which usually meant working from six 'till ten. I heard nothing, and after six weeks I assumed that there were no vacancies, but what the heck. I decided to phone up and ask any-way. Well, you could have knocked me down with a feather when I was told that I was due to start that night, as I had already been added to the off duty. I hastily explained that as no one had informed me, I would have to start tomorrow night instead. I didn't tell them that I still hadn't told my husband. I was asked if I could work from eight o'clock until midnight instead of six 'till ten. That worked out better still, the children would be in bed, and I would have time for a sit down and a cup of tea before starting my shift.

When Ray came home from work, I waited until after dinner when the children were in bed, and then I casually asked,

"What do you think about me going back to work?"

"How could you with two kids to look after?" he replied.

"I've been thinking", I said. "What if I worked the six 'till ten shift?"

"If you think you could do it, it's up to you", he said.

"Oh, good", I said. "I start tomorrow, except it's been changed to eight 'till midnight".

"What? You've got it all arranged? When did you do that?"

He didn't really mind, but the next day was quite hectic as I had to get to the hospital to be measured for my very first staff nurses' uniform. Luckily, uniforms were all kept in stock in a variety of sizes, and all that needed to be done was to sew the hem at the right length. I was asked if I wanted long or short-sleeved dresses. If I had the long sleeved, I would have to have cuffs as well, but I plumped for the short sleeves. That evening as I went to work, I was both excited and apprehensive, like starting out on my first day all over again. All my uniforms, dresses, aprons, caps, and belts had been left out for me. I got changed and looked in the mirror, and for the very first time there, looking back at me, was a proper staff nurse. I hurried along to the night sisters' office to report for duty and to be allocated to a ward. I couldn't believe my ears when I was told that I would be working in casualty. It felt like I had won the pools, and that's where I worked for the next twenty-four years.

CHAPTER TEN

I made my way down to casualty, my heart in my mouth. I was praying that I wouldn't be left on my own. After all, I hadn't practised any kind of nursing, let alone been a staff nurse, for two and a half years. I put on my most confident face, smoothed down my already smooth apron, and walked confidently into 'cas'. I was given a lightning tour of where everything was kept, and then all the day staff left at nine o'clock. That left me and one other staff nurse who worked the granny shift and was due to finish at ten. I was practically wetting myself. They couldn't seriously leave me on my own. Margaret was very good and assured me that I would be fine. She stayed late, chatting to me and showing me the paper work. At night there was no receptionist or office staff, so the nurse had to do it all, starting with registering the patient and making out a casualty card – the job that 'Blondie' used to do in the record office when I was a cadet. But the scary bit was the fact that the doctor was not actually in the casualty. They stayed in the doctors' house and only came over for the more serious injuries. The only good thing about this system was that the doctors were only to keen to teach me how to check for injuries, how to stitch the more simple lacerations, and how to check for broken bones, so I learned a lot. For the most part, there were no regular casualty doctors, and they were not keen on being called over. They would invariably say that if the patient was brought back the next day to be seen, everything would be fine.

There were many ups and downs working on your own at night. The only other people around were the switchboard operator and the porter, who would sit with the telephonist once his work was done. There was only one telephonist at a time who worked nights. One of them was blind, and he would feel his way around the keys. He was so quick that no one would have guessed he couldn't see. I also found out pretty soon that when it was very busy, no one seemed to like coming down to help. Apparently, before I started they had tried for a long time to get someone to work nights in casualty but no one would.

Over the next few years, there were many memorable incidents. I nearly split my sides laughing the night a man presented at casualty to announce that he thought he had rabies. He had come straight from the airport, complete with luggage. He had just returned from a holiday in Africa, and before leaving he had been bitten by a dog. Now I know that none of that is funny. What was funny was when I reported it all to the night sister. There were four night sisters, and the one who was in charge that night went into overdrive.

"Don't tell anyone", she said. "We don't want to start a panic. Get the wall washers in and tell them to burn anything that can be burnt. They've got to wash everything. And don't say a word".

Well, I thought she was kidding, but she was deadly serious, and she was not impressed by the fact that I was treating the whole episode less seriously than she was. I tried to reason with her through my giggles, but she was having none of it. So when the wall washers put in an appearance, they not surprisingly asked what it was they were handling. My lips were sealed. They went away and reappeared some half an hour later, looking like they were going to the moon. All that was visible was their eyes, which could just be seen through their goggles. True to their instructions, casualty had been duly stripped of all the stretcher covers, pillows, curtains, blankets, sheets – you name it. If it would go in the incinerator, that's were it went. It took all of my persuasive powers to stop them from burning all the patients' notes as well. By now I reckoned that this had gone too far, and I found the night sister to tell her so. I tried to explain that you couldn't just catch rabies. You would have to be bitten at the very least by an animal that had rabies, but she was having none of it. The wall washers had to continue their job, thinking they were handling something highly contagious – a plague at the very least. I would have given my right arm to be a fly on the wall when the staff arrived the next day to a casualty that had been totally stripped bare. Mind you, I had a pretty good idea, because the next night when I went to work, the place was still bare. Everyone was waiting for me. They wanted to know what was going on. Where was everything? The linen room ladies were going mad. The rumour had gone round the hospital that all the linen had been burnt, but they couldn't believe it.

"Couldn't you stop her?" they asked.

"I did try". I explained what had happened. You just couldn't make it up, something like that.

I worked four nights a week, from eight o'clock until midnight. I had been working for several months when it occurred to me that I should be getting the night allowance, so I duly went along to night sisters' office and put it to her that I was under the night staff and therefore I should be receiving the allowance.

"No, you shouldn't. You have to work the whole night to get that", she told me.

"I'll phone salaries and wages and ask them", I said.

"No you won't, staff nurse. I've told you you're not entitled to it".

But I thought she was wrong, and true to form I resolved to find out. The next day I phoned salaries and wages. Of course I should be getting a night allowance; the mistake was all theirs. Although I had filled out my time sheets, putting the A.M. and the P.M. in the correct place, they just assumed I was repeatedly making the same mistake and they changed them. I was the only one in the whole hospital working these hours. They apologised, and I got a nice bit of back pay the following week. Strangely, the night sister was not too happy. She was noticeable narked that I did not take her word for it that I was not entitled to the allowance. As my senior, she felt I should have accepted what she said, but why change the habit of a lifetime. She made the comment,

"You decided to phone wages anyway, did you".
"Yes", I said lightly. "I thought it was worth a try".

It certainly was; the night allowance on sixteen hours made a big difference.

Gradually, I became more confident working on my own at night in casualty. The only thing I dreaded was when the red phone rang. That phone was the hot line – a direct link to ambulance control to tell me if a patient was coming in with life-threatening injuries or a cardiac arrest. I would get a few minutes to get things prepared and to get a doctor over. Injuries, no matter how severe, I could handle confidently, but cardiac arrest took me a long time to get the same level of confidence.

For the next couple of years, things jogged along quite nicely. I loved the work I was doing, and the hours I worked meant that I didn't have to rely on baby sitters, and life was pretty good.

Barrow, as well as heavy industry, also had docks, cargo mostly, and when they closed down, my dad, who was a docker, got a job as an ambulance driver. First he drove the carriers – the vehicles that were used to transport patients to the hospital for appointments, or those who were being transferred to other hospitals. Then he went onto shift work, driving the emergency vehicles.

Now everyone who has ever worked in a casualty, even back in the sixties or seventies, knew that some patients were habitual 'attendees', even if there was nothing wrong with them. Some of our regulars used the ambulance as a taxi service. Nine times out of ten, they fitted the same category of being young, male, and drunk. North Lonsdale being in the middle of town meant that it was in a very convenient location for a dropping off place, especially late at night. These time wasters, usually the same people over and over again, after being brought to the hospital would get out of the back of the ambulance and then leg it, shouting,

"Thanks for the lift, mate".

I have to admit that these people were infuriating. My dad didn't like being taken for a mug, and he was no taxi driver, so when he was working with certain like-minded ambulance drivers – in particular one Alan Simpson – between them they decided to teach some of the regulars a lesson. As a result, these drunks found themselves being dumped up the Woods Road or Mill Wood or down the Coast Road – basically about two or three miles from the town centre. The first few 'patients' couldn't believe what was happening when the back doors were opened and they were kicked out, and they realised they had a long walk home. Luckily, mobiles hadn't been invented, so they couldn't just call for another ambulance. Word soon spread, and the number of inappropriate 999 calls dropped right down.

These young males were no different to today's mouthy youths, and one Saturday night we had more than our fair share of troublemakers. You know the kind of thing:

"Hey, you, see to me. I want to get home. I pay your wages", mixed in with expletives and swearing. One Saturday night, my dad had had enough. The drunk in the back of his ambulance was mouthing off from the minute he got in. Dad sat there and never said a word while he, the so-called patient, called him all the names under the sun. But it was at the point when he said,

"You have to take me to hospital "cause you're f-ing paid to".

The F word was not in common use then and to use it was considered to be highly insulting.

That was it. He pushed one button to many. Dad told the driver to pull over.

"You're f-ing bluffing", continued the inebriate. "You wouldn't dare".

Oh yes he would, and Dad opened the back doors of the ambulance and told him to get out or be kicked out. He got out of his own accord and he was left standing in the road, shouting and swearing as the ambulance drove away.

"I'm going to complain about you", he shouted after the fast-disappearing ambulance, but he didn't.

Very occasionally, if someone had been abusive in casualty, they did return the next day to apologise, but it didn't happen that often.

There was also a time when my dad sat patiently listening to the man who was being sectioned under the mental health act, who was being transported to Ridge Lea at Lancaster. My dad could be a good listener, and at times like these, he just listened, nodded his head occasionally, and agreed with whatever the man was saying. The man seemed quite calm, so it came as quite a shock when Dad said,

"Not long now, mate. We're nearly there".

With that, the man got up and said,

"I'll be off, then",

and he tried to open the back doors of the ambulance while it was going at seventy miles an hour down the motorway. Dad had to wrestle with him to get him away from the doors and talk quickly to convince him that opening the doors was not a good idea. Eventually, he got him back to his seat and calmed him down again.

I worked these hours quite happily for several years before switching to part-time days. Actually, days were pretty good because there were other nurses to get opinions from, and there were all the back up services, such as x-ray and path lab – no more waiting for on call to come in. It took a bit of getting use to, that I didn't have to do everything myself, but the biggest thing to get used to was the hustle and bustle of so many people being around.

Gradually, more and more guidelines were introduced and there were more tasks that had to be taken into consideration, bearing in mind that the area had a lot of heavy industry and Glaxos Pharmaceutical company was just a short distance away. Procedures had to be put in place on how to handle a major accident.

Equipment was duly ordered, and when it arrived there was so much that we had to be allocated a large storeroom to keep it all in. We were told to familiarise ourselves with all the stuff and how to use it. As well as how to pack it so that we knew exactly where to find each individual item. To go along with all this was some top-quality, all-weather gear. You name it and it had been provided. We were also told to get ourselves prepared because a large mock major accident was being arranged to include all the services, and there would be only a few minutes warning.

The call came through a few weeks later, when the initial curiosity and excitement over the new equipment had worn off, and we had all been lulled into a false sense of security. Thank goodness we had all been to acquaint ourselves with the paraphernalia. It was in the morning that the plan was put into operation. A call came through from ambulance control that the major accident plan was being implemented. Guess who was told they were to accompany the doctor? Little old me. I was looking forward to this, but at the same time I was also nervous. In fact, the first thing I had to do was to go running to the toilet.

It was actually a nice day. The sun was shining, and it was nice and warm. It couldn't have been better. I got all my gear on, including the day glow bib with 'nurse' written across the back. I could have climbed Mount Everest in that lot. It was a good job I was young and fit because when I swung the haversack onto my back, the weight of it nearly knocked me over. I actually staggered several paces sideways like a crab before I got my balance back.

We were joined by the nurses from the wards who had been allocated to help, and then we waited, and we waited, and then it dawned on us that we didn't know how we were supposed to get there. We had assumed that an ambulance would come, but it didn't. It had raced off without us. Oh, dear. Well, that's what these exercises were all about: to iron out any little hiccups. Eventually it was decided that we would share the ambulance that had been sent to take all the supplies to the scene, but there wasn't enough room for us, so we kind of squashed up all on one side because one of the stretchers had been removed to make more room for the equipment. It was all very cosy with our feet on top of our rucksacks and our arms holding onto sacks full of bandages and such. We almost disappeared under a sea of bags.

We were taken to the Walney aerodrome where this huge mock up had been staged. We got out of the ambulance and were confronted with bodies everywhere and people shouting and crying. Blimey, the local Am. Dram group was having a field day. They were covered in fake blood and dirt; it was very realistic. For a moment, we kind of just stood there taking it all in. I was thinking,

"Where the hell do I start?"

Our job was to assess the casualties and tag them with a number according to how severe the injuries were, and get the most severe off to hospital first. I was actually the only one who knew how the number system worked; the nurses from the ward didn't have a clue, and the doctor, who was a local G.P., didn't know either. So, I gave them a crash course on the way while we were travelling to the scene.

I sprang into action – super nurse to the rescue – and I ran over to the first person I could see. Well, actually that's a lie because I couldn't run anywhere with the weight of the huge backpack I had to carry. Now I know how a tortoise feels carrying the weight of its house on its back. The first thing you do when confronted with an unconscious casualty is check whether they are breathing and whether they have a pulse. Obviously everyone was breathing and they all had a pulse on account of them only acting, so how the heck was I to know that the very first patient I went to was playing dead. No one had told us that we were to check their pockets for a little card that said 'DEAD'. This patient certainly wasn't talking to me, so after spending quite some time with him, I was about to immobilise what appeared to be a fractured femur, when he opened his eyes and whispered,

"There's a card in me pocket, nurse".

I didn't know what he was on about, but I looked anyway, and there it was: the word 'DEAD' printed on a little card. He could have told me sooner, but I think he was enjoying the attention.

We were there for hours until eventually the last casualty had been taken to hospital. By this time, the poor doctor was bursting for a pee. I kept seeing the men going into the bushes. At first I wondered if there were hidden casualties, and I was just about to investigate when the doc said,

"I wouldn't, if I were you. I'm going to go there myself".

And he explained what they were all doing, I felt really stupid for not realising.

Sorry for mentioning that, doc, but if ever you read this, you will know instantly who you are. After that, every time he saw me he remembered the incident when he had had to go into the bushes for a pee. Needs must, I suppose, be met, whereas the nurses just had to cross their legs and hope they would get back in time before their bladders had burst. We packed up the gear and returned exhausted, thirsty, and hungry to casualty. There were a lot of lessons to be learned, and it was an exercise well worth doing.

The G.P.s worked on a regular basis in casualty, covering about half of the shifts. All the doctors from one practise took it in turns to provide cover, hence the reason why it was a G.P. who went out to the mock up. Hospital doctors only provided cover, but no one actually specialised in casualty.

CHAPTER ELEVEN

Over the years many changes took place, including the closure of all the small local hospitals: Roose gynaecology with its thirty beds, although for the time being the Roose geriatric hospital would stay open and the central laundry would stay there; The Devonshire Road Children's; High Carley; and of course North Lonsdale Hospital. Things were never the same again once the Furness General Hospital opened in October 1984 and all the others ceased to exist. All the old hospitals have since been demolished and housing estates have been built in their place, except for the North Lonsdale and Risedale hospitals, where they built nursing homes. Going from lots of small hospitals where everyone knew each other to one big hospital were half the staff were strangers took a bit of getting use to.

I think it was at this point that we lost the matrons in favour of nurse managers. Now call me nostalgic if you like, but I think that this was the start of the N.H.S. going ever so slightly downhill, especially as they didn't even wear a uniform – they were in mufti. In my opinion, it was the uniform that carried respect.

None the less this was progress. At long last we had the new hospital that the area had been promised for the last thirty years. Except that this one was so big we could have done with motor scooters to get around on, compared with what we were used to, that is. With the new hospital came new technology and new ways of doing things. The first hurdle to overcome was the fact that no one had spotted that the telephone exchange was scheduled to be built in phase two not phase one of the building. One of the X-ray rooms was hastily allocated to house the new exchange. That caused its own problems, as the room was lead lined. Eventually a relay system was fitted so that the phones would work.

The hospital was situated on a thirty-five-acre site on the edge of town, right next to Monks Croft and Priors Lea, which also sported a helicopter pad on the grounds. This caused quite a stir of excitement, as new guidelines had to be drawn up to meet any incoming helicopters. It was like something out of M.A.S.H. Imaginations went into overdrive. Being right on the edge of the Lake District, there were a fair number of casualties who fell off mountains or hurt themselves in a variety of ways, quite often by preparing to climb a mountain while wearing such things as flip-flops and dressed for a summer"s out-ing. They were invariably taken by surprise when the weather would suddenly change, when what might start out as a sunny day would suddenly turn wet and cold. You'd be surprised by how many people don't realise that the air is colder higher up the mountain they had managed to climb, and flip flops are not the best footwear on loose shingle. Anyway, there were times when the helicopter was used to bring casualties in – a journey that would take a few minutes compared to a tortuous route by road.

When the helicopters first started coming, there was no shortage of volunteers to go over and meet them. There would also be the police, who had to shut the road during landing, the fire service, which had to attend in case of any mishap, and of course the ambulance to transport the patient. For anyone who has never been in close proximity to the whirling blades of a landing helicopter, let me describe it for you.

First, everyone stands around with their eyes gazing upwards to see who is the first to spot the 'copter, and then you would hear the yell,

"Here it comes".

Then all eyes would turn to follow the outstretched finger pointing up into the sky to a tiny dot a long way off. Gradually as it got closer, you would hear the noise getting louder and louder, until eventually you couldn't hear yourself speak and you had to cover your ears to avoid burst eardrums. Then as this big machine circles round to come into land, it would be as though you were in the middle of a tornado, or at the very least a severe gale-force wind.

There was never a need to sweep the surrounding paths because one of these things landing sent all the dirt flying into oblivion. Not only that, all the trees and shrubs, especially in the autumn would be suddenly stripped of all their leaves. Yes, girls, you hung onto your dress for dear life if you wanted to preserve your modesty, and forget your hair, because it would be blown straight out, whatever style it started off in. And always remember to remove your cap, because it does not stay on your head for very long. Add to all that, say, driving rain or freezing cold, and suddenly helicopters landing don't seem quite so exciting as they use to. Eventually we had a kind of one-walled bus shelter put up so that we could be a little protected, but as soon as the ambulance arrived we could sit in that. After all, there is only the nurse and doctor who arrive on foot after running through the hospital, casualty being on the opposite side to the heli-pad. Everyone else comes in their own transport.

It brings to mind one occasion not long after they had started using the big Sea King helicopters – they were a sight worth seeing. These huge yellow things created twice the down draught of anything previously used. So there we all were one afternoon. It was actually sunny, sitting in the back of the ambulance. We waited outside until the helicopter got close, and then we dived into the sanctuary of the ambulance, waiting to hear the by now familiar sound of the rotor blades. The Barrow fire brigade must have been busy, and a fire tender from the small town up the road had been dispatched to do the honours. As we looked out of the window, we watched as the firemen got out and duly pulled out the hoses and laid them in neat rows on the ground.

"I hope they're not expecting to use them", someone said wryly.

We thought it a bit strange, as no one else had ever done this, but they weren't finished yet. They next all lined up in front of their lovely clean fire truck for a photo opportunity just as the helicopter started to land. As far as I was aware, this was the first time they had sent a fire engine from another station. I don't know if they ever got their photo. They all looked so proud as they stood to attention, waiting to catch the helicopter and their fire engine in the same shot. Alas, it didn't quite work out. At first the hoses took on a mind of their own as the downdraught kicked in, but then one by one the firemans helmets blew off and rolled down the slope and far away. Trumpton came to mind as they all set off to retrieve them, running as the helmets gathered pace, helped along by the terrific wind that the blades caused. Sorry, lads, but I laughed 'till the tears ran down my face. I'm sorry to say I laughed every time I retold the tale. In fact, I could hardly tell it for laughing. The poor patient must have wondered what on earth was going on, but he was taken safely to the casualty.

There are so many things that happen in casualty, but one of the memorable things I just have to include is something I'll never forget. It is the story of an elderly lady brought to casualty, which by now had had a name change and was known as accident and emergency. She was brought in late one evening. The poor thing was so distressed she was positively wailing.

"What about me little doggy", she cried. "He's in the house all on his own. He's all I've got. My only friend. He"s company for me".

She was so upset that I was nearly crying with her. I"ve always been a sucker for animals, so I thought I would ask a young constable who was in casualty at the time if there was anything he could do to help. He said he would try, and he set off for the lady's address on his motorbike. He phoned me to tell me it would not be easy to get the dog into kennels, as it had not had its injections. Eventually he found kennels with an isolation area. I don't know how he got the little terrier to the kennels, but he did.

Meanwhile, I started to undress the lady to get her ready for the doctor to examine her. She was wearing a very obvious wig, which I left undisturbed so as not to embarrass her. As I undressed her, money started falling out from her clothing. It was up her sleeves, in her bra, and down her knickers. In fact, money had been stuffed everywhere – more than two thousand pounds of it. In her handbag were at least half a dozen bank books with deposits of thousands of pounds.

Eventually the policeman came back, pleased that he had found somewhere for the dog, and he told the lady how hard it had been because the dog wasn't vaccinated. She was so grateful.

"Thank you so much, dear", she said. "He's my only friend. I"m ever so grateful".

The young policeman said,

"I'm glad I could help, and it's only a pound a night".

The lady nearly had a heart attack.

"A pound a night?" she said. "I can't afford that. I'm a pensioner. You'll have to get it put down".

Her tears stopped instantly. We just looked at each other in disbelief. The constable told me that her house had money in every drawer. There were several thousand pounds scattered all over. I told

him how much money I had found in her clothing. When I took her to the ward, I told them the
tale of the dog and the money. Some time later, the
ward phoned down to tell me they'd removed the
wig at the patient's request, only to find five hundred
pounds sitting on her head. I don't know what happened to the dog or if she ever paid the kennel fees.
She may have pleaded poverty and got the boarding
for free, but I know the dog wasn't put down.

Then there were the smart alecks. One man came
in with his mother and promptly told me what treatment she needed.

"I know what's wrong with her", he said, "because my wife is a nurse".

Without batting an eyelid I said,

"My husband's a joiner, but I can't make a window".

There are many tales I could tell, some of them
funny, and some of them sad, but maybe I'll save
them for another day.

Looking back over the decades, I think back to
the sixties when the National Health Service was
still riding very much on the crest of a wave. It was
admired around the world. The population on the
whole treated it with respect, especially older people who knew what it was like to be sick when they
could not afford a doctor. Working in the N.H.S.
was something to be proud of then. Now I am not

so sure. People demand so much from our N.H.S., such as the man who came to casualty one Christmas Day with what he described as an abscess, though I would have said it was no more than a large spot. I asked him what made him come on Christmas Day when the spot had obviously been there for some time.

"I was just passing", he said, "so I thought I would call in".

Then there was the man who had literally cut himself shaving who called in for a plaster because he was going out. What happened to the piece of tissue men usually stick on their faces when they cut themselves shaving? There are many people who should have gone to a G.P., but who couldn't be bothered to make an appointment, so they called at the casualty instead. There is also a new breed of patient who now look up their symptoms on the Internet. They present their own diagnoses, along with a list of treatments they want. No, not want – more like demand.

I would say that all these types of people abuse the N.H.S., and that is a shame because the concept behind it is very laudable. If things continue as they are, we will all wake up one day and the National Health Service will have ceased to exist. I think there are lots of things we could do to stop the rot, but for once, I'll keep my mouth shut.

Lightning Source UK Ltd.
Milton Keynes UK
29 April 2010

153505UK00001B/21/P